# cinch!

# cinch!

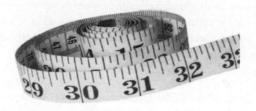

## conquer cravings, drop pounds, and lose inches

# Cynthia Sass, MPH, RD

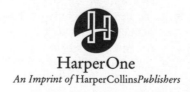

HarperOne
*An Imprint of* HarperCollins*Publishers*

HarperOne

CINCH! *Conquer Cravings, Drop Pounds, and Lose Inches.* Copyright © 2010 by Cynthia Sass. All rights reserved. Printed in the United States of America. No part of this book may be used or reproduced in any manner whatsoever without written permission except in the case of brief quotations embodied in critical articles and reviews. For information address HarperCollins Publishers, 10 East 53rd Street, New York, NY 10022.

HarperCollins books may be purchased for educational, business, or sales promotional use. For information please write: Special Markets Department, HarperCollins Publishers, 10 East 53rd Street, New York, NY 10022.

HarperCollins website: http://www.harpercollins.com

HarperCollins®, 📖 ®, and HarperOne™ are trademarks of HarperCollins Publishers.

FIRST EDITION

*Designed by Nicola Ferguson*
*Interior photography © Chad Tenorio*

Library of Congress Cataloging-in-Publication Data
Sass, Cynthia.
Cinch! : conquer cravings, drop pounds, and lose inches / Cynthia Sass. — 1st ed.
p. cm.
ISBN 978–0–06–197464–9
1. Reducing diets. 2. Weight loss. I. Title.
RM222.2.S2515 2011
613.2'5—dc22
2010027066

10  11  12  13  14   RRD(H)   10  9  8  7  6  5  4  3  2  1

*For Jack Bremen and Diane Salvagno, my two lifelines*
*and lifesavers!*

# contents

Introduction    *1*

1. The Cinch! Plan: Freedom from Diet Chaos    *9*

2. The 5-Day, 5-Food Fast Forward    *28*

3. A Little SASS Goes a Long Way    *70*

4. The Cinch! Core    *90*

5. Your Daily Chocolate Escape    *137*

6. The Do-It-Yourself 5-Piece Puzzle    *149*

7. Losing Is a Cinch!    *188*

8. Conquer Emotional Eating    *213*

9. Fall in Love with Walking    *235*

10. Just in Case You Asked . . .    *249*

11. Cinch! Goes the Distance    *268*

Acknowledgments    *283*

Index    *285*

About the Author    *295*

# introduction

Over the years I've helped countless people, especially women, experience what I call "Yes!" moments. Maybe you've been longing for one yourself: The zipper on your skinny jeans slides up effortlessly; you discover that you can wear a clingy dress or skirt *without* Spanx; you walk down the beach or slide into the pool free from a cover-up or oversize tee; you don't panic and reach for a towel when your husband walks in on you getting out of the shower.

Every time one of my clients recounts a "Yes!" event with me, I get goose bumps, because the confidence and bliss people radiate when they've achieved weight-loss success is electric. A moment like that can keep you on an emotional high for days, and helping someone bask in that glow of self-confidence is one of the reasons I love my job.

This book is going to help you achieve more than one "Yes!" moment.

The first will come after just five days, when you have completed my 5-Food Fast Forward program. The second will
come twenty-five days later, when you've graduated from
Cinch! core, a plan that includes four delicious, perfectly
proportioned quick-fix meals per day—how does Peanut
Butter Blackberry Toast sound for breakfast? And there
is a *mandatory* daily dark-chocolate escape. That's right—
chocolate *every day*. But even more important, this book
will prime you for countless future moments of body satisfaction because the weight-loss method you'll uncover in
these pages holds the power to transform your life. At the
end of these thirty days, you'll feel as if a switch has been
flipped that can never be shut off. You'll relate to food and
your body in an entirely new way, one that won't allow you to return to the
eating chaos that led you to pick up this book.

Okay, so you're probably wondering, What exactly am I going to
be eating? Here's how my plan works: During the Fast Forward stage,
you'll eat just five foods in various combinations: spinach, almonds,
raspberries, eggs, and yogurt, or vegan-friendly alternatives. These
foods represent the purest form of a clean-eating plan. Each food was
carefully chosen because of its natural detoxifying nutrients as well as
emerging evidence of its weight-loss power. These first five days will give
your body, mind, and taste buds a clean slate and help you lose weight
healthfully while providing energy and nourishment. And, you'll lose
weight fast. The exactness of the 5-Day Fast Forward provides its power.
The Fast Forward allows you to lose up to eight pounds in just five days,
and its challenge empowers you to easily transition to the twenty-five-
day Cinch! core plan that will keep you losing! Once you learn how
easy it is to lose on Cinch!, you'll have all the tools you need to keep
losing, or if you've reached your goal weight, to embrace a lifelong pattern of healthful eating.

Losing weight is now a cinch! All you need to do each day to achieve
your weight-loss goal is:

1. Look through the meal lists.
2. Choose any breakfast, lunch, dinner, and snack meal you like.
3. Make the meals exactly as stated.
4. Eat your first meal within one hour of waking up and enjoy the remaining meals three to five hours apart.

At no point will you count calories. The emphasis during both the Fast Forward and throughout Cinch! core is on meal timing, portions, combinations of foods, and food quality. This plan is specifically designed to help you lose body fat from head to toe, optimize your health, transform your emotional relationship with food and your body, and give you the tools to successfully take the weight off!

According to a Johns Hopkins study, by the year 2015, 75 percent of adults in the United States will be overweight, and 41 percent will qualify as obese. By comparison, in 1996, 34 percent of U.S. adults were overweight and 17 percent were obese. The plain truth is, we've been programmed to eat when food is available and use food as a tool to cope with our emotional needs. It is easy to live a lifestyle where you overeat, day after day, week after week, month after month, year after year.

But when you change your relationship with food, as this book will show you how, you can change the way you eat and, as a result, change your body.

## wait, what about *flat belly diet!*?

If you're a fan of *Flat Belly Diet!*, for which I created the eating plan in 2007, you may wonder, Why am I promoting a new plan, and how is this one different?

The field of nutrition is ever changing. Since *Flat Belly Diet!* was published, my philosophies have been enhanced by a wealth of new research. I've attended scientific conferences, counseled many more people, and traveled to other parts of the world to study nutrition and public health. In this book, I combine some of the research I used to develop the *Flat Belly Diet!* eating plan with new studies, fresh insights, added wisdom, and exciting emerging information about how to lose weight and keep it off.

### What's Similar? Cinch! Also

- Emphasizes a Mediterranean-style eating plan with produce, whole grains, lean protein, and healthy fats, including MUFAs (monounsaturated fats)
- Provides lists of quick and easy meals you can make as described
- Provides interchangeable meals: in Flat Belly Diet!, all of the meals were interchangeable; in this plan, breakfasts and snacks are interchangeable and lunch and dinner meals are interchangeable

### What's Different? Cinch!

- Emphasizes portions and balance instead of calorie counts
- Places a much stronger emphasis on whole foods and local and organic foods
- Ensures that you get a specific number of servings from each food group each day, including two fruit and four veggie servings
- Lets you customize the size of your meals to your body's needs
- Actually insists on a daily dark-chocolate indulgence!
- Offers coconut oil as a good-for-you fat option with yummy recipes featuring this tasty oil
- Is vegetarian- and vegan-friendly and recommends more plant-based meals
- Includes specific guidelines for water and other beverages
- Incorporates powerful SASS, Slimming And Satiating Seasonings, at every meal
- Offers a meal-building "puzzle" that teaches you to create your own Cinch!-friendly meals at home or away from home

Overall, this plan features fresh, whole, natural, unprocessed, and organic foods to help you quickly and efficiently achieve the body of your dreams. I designed the meals to provide the very best nutrients for your body with the perfect balance of carbohydrates, protein, and "good" fat—to keep you fuller longer, better control your blood sugar and insulin levels, and delay the return of hunger.

You'll also learn to take charge of your eating so that you don't need to rely on me. Within one month, instead of feeling overwhelmed when you walk down the bread aisle at the supermarket, perhaps wondering if you should even eat bread, you'll feel completely confident about which bread to buy and why, how to eat it, what to eat it with, how much to have, and how often. You'll be able to visualize precisely how to put meals together, whether at home or at a restaurant—meals that are satisfying, nourishing, and delicious and make you feel amazing inside and out. Meals that will help you reach your goal weight and then easily stay there!

In a nutshell, if you follow the plan I provide in the pages to come, here's what you'll achieve:

- Weight loss—up to 8 pounds in the first 5 days
- Increased self-confidence
- Mastery of the tactics proven to keep weight off
- An understanding of the powerful emotions that drive you to eat when you're not hungry
- Better health, including a surge in energy; enhanced disease protection; antiaging benefits; better immunity, digestion, and sleep; better-looking skin and hair; and fewer mood swings

You won't have to give up your morning cup of coffee, forego chocolate or peanut butter, start an exercise plan today, stop dining out, spend hours in the kitchen, give up carbs, or eat skimpy portions. My clients who have followed this plan unanimously tell me: Wow, this is totally doable! You'll find comments and success stories from Cinch! enthusiasts throughout the book.

## what sets this plan apart

Chances are you've lost weight in the past. Over the years, maybe you've even had some exciting "Yes!" moments but for a handful of reasons wound up right back where you started—or possibly even five steps behind. I've met hundreds of women, and men, who have dieted themselves from single- to double-digit sizes and are stuck in a vicious cycle of losing twenty pounds, gaining back twenty-five, losing thirty, gaining back thirty-eight. I understand why that happens, and in this book, I'm going to help you break that cycle.

That's one of the important ways this book is different from any other "diet" book on the shelf. This plan isn't about following an imposed set of rules that don't really make sense or don't intuitively feel nourishing. It's about truly understanding how your body works and what it needs, and eating in a way that honors the body-mind connection you were born with—the one that got caught in chaos throughout the years. This plan will not only give you results; it will connect the "what," "when," "how," and "why" aspects of eating in a way that becomes crystal clear like nothing has before. You'll gain both confidence and a sense of food freedom that will transform how you look and feel—forever.

## lose weight and conquer emotional eating

When I was growing up, I had strong influences that led me to become a nutritionist and health educator. One of these was witnessing constant diet chaos. Most of the women in my life lived in a continual cycle of being "on" or "off" myriad crazy diets. "On" meant being "good," restricting— not enjoying—food, looking and feeling weak, and applying "willpower." "Off" meant overeating forbidden food and treats and a short-term sense of fun and freedom followed by impending guilt, rebound weight gain, self-berating comments, and depression.

My goal is to help you see food as a means of achieving weight-loss success that doesn't require self-sacrifice. I want you to view food as a way of nourishing and taking care of the most precious resource you have: you! At the end of every meal, I want you to feel full (but not overly full), satisfied, energized, nourished, and ready to move on with your day without continuing to think about eating. I want you to feel like you have the energy to do cartwheels down the street and feel a sense of pride and confidence about your relationship with food, and I want you to have the body you've always wanted!

## end diet chaos starting today

You can't control many of the things that impact your life, but you *can* control your relationship with your body—and that means you can control your weight, how you feel, and, to a large extent, your health. That's why this thirty-day program is life changing. No matter what else is going on, taking charge of your body makes you feel like you can conquer the world.

Successfully losing weight and changing how and why you eat is so empowering that it impacts not only how you feel physically and emotionally, but also how you interact with others and how you react in any given situation. When you feel great about you—inside and out—you radiate a different energy and navigate the world in an entirely different way, at work, with your friends and family, even waiting in line at the post office. Losing weight healthfully creates a domino effect that alters your body language and the way you hold yourself, how you dress, how you walk, and how you feel about all of the other aspects of self-caretaking. By the end of this thirty-day program, you will not only shed pounds and inches but you will gain a sense of confidence and strength that transcends every aspect of your life. While you will see both immediate and lasting change, you'll also be delighted by your daily experience of eating delicious meals, savoring a daily chocolate treat, and embracing new tastes. Losing weight really is a cinch!

# 1

`24 25 26 27 28 29 30 31 32 33`

# the cinch! plan

## freedom from diet chaos

Cinch! is the catalyst you've been waiting for—the simple plan that makes you think, "Yes, I can do this!" I've laid out a concise prescription that, in just thirty days, has the power to profoundly change the way you look and feel, and free you from diet chaos.

By "diet chaos," I mean the erratic eating cycle most dieters find they've been trapped in for years, if not decades. Nearly everyone I meet who struggles with weight issues has fallen into a similar pattern, and chances are you're right there, too. Do you find that everything related to your diet is inconsistent, from your food and drink choices to how much and how often you eat? Some days, you may be so distracted that you end up squeezing in just one solid meal, relying mostly on sporadic, unhealthy snacks—an energy bar here, a diet soda and crackers there. Then other days feel like an all-day Las Vegas buffet.

Perhaps your emotions are so intertwined with your eating that food has become like a drug. Have you ever turned to chips or cookies to combat the boredom and stress of caring for young children or an aging parent or to escape the grind of work, bills, and household chores? Or maybe you look to food as a reward. I counsel a lot of working moms who give, give, give, and then feel—understandably—that they deserve something special in return. But all too often, their "gift" to themselves turns out to be a big bowl of ice cream—and extra pounds on their thighs. Other people munch because there's a big box of chocolate crullers in their office break room or simply because it's dinnertime, even if they're not hungry.

When your pattern is that you have no pattern, it's impossible to know when you are hungry or full. So, at times you end up eating less than your body needs, which triggers a metabolism slowdown to conserve energy. At other times you overeat, so excess calories get socked away in your fat cells. Your energy slumps, and you become irritable: you might find yourself fighting with your partner over who forgot to take out the recycling. Depression, anxiety, and either weight gain or, at least, failure to lose weight aren't uncommon under these circumstances, and constipation and water retention are almost inevitable.

There's only one answer to this kind of diet chaos: order. That's what Cinch! offers, but you won't feel like you're in reform school or diet boot camp. This plan is based on a set of *simple,* inspiring, doable steps that will guide you in building confidence and learning to eat in a way that becomes intuitive and liberating! The main reason you need structure—starting today—is that your body thrives on balance and consistency. With Cinch! you'll quickly come to understand what stability feels like. And as a result, you'll reshape your body and feel amazing inside and out. But best of all, you'll lose weight without having to count calories or grams of fat, carbs, or sugar, or memorize complex charts. In the pages to come you'll learn the clear-cut, sustainable secrets to weight-loss success so you can get your body back and redirect your energy to where it should be flowing—toward living and enjoying your life.

## the plan in a nutshell

Rules are the foundation of change; they create boundaries that prevent you from feeling overwhelmed and guidelines to keep you on track. In a nutshell, rules make changing your diet a cinch! By following the set I've laid out, you'll know exactly what to do, but more important, you'll also learn by doing. It's a lot like learning to drive. You can observe as a passenger and take a driver's education class, but you never really master control until you're the one behind the wheel; then, with a little experience, it all becomes effortless.

Chapters 4 and 6 explain the rules in much more detail and include the actual eating plans, but here are the basics: Cinch! is a thirty-day plan that offers a 5-Day, 5-Food Fast Forward option that jump-starts your results. The 5-Day Fast Forward isn't for everyone, nor is it necessary for achieving terrific weight-loss results. But if you're the type of person who thrives on quick results, I'm sure you'll love it. To decide whether you're a good candidate for the Fast Forward, take the quiz on page 16.

The core of Cinch!—the twenty-five-day plan—will help you make profound changes to your way of eating that are easily doable and amazingly rewarding. You will eliminate processed foods and artificial additives—say good-bye to those frozen dinners and hello to a slimmer you—while enjoying the enticing flavors of wholesome, natural foods, from juicy in-season fruits and hearty whole grains to decadent nut butters and a daily dose of dark chocolate. And I give you all the tools, tips, and tricks to make these meals just as convenient as reaching for a bag of chips. Here's what you'll eat: four simple, luscious meals a day, each made from nutrient-packed, clean, whole foods you'll feel virtuous about eating. The power of the plan is in the foods that make up your four daily meals. (And you'll find a daily decadent treat that you'll

> 24 25 26 27 28 29 30
>
> Feeling a bit lighter after two days. My body is happier; no heavy feeling in the morning.
> CHRIS, AGE 54

look forward to every day.) My plan is based on cutting-edge research and three key rules that work in synergy to give you real and lasting results:

**Rule 1: Eat Like Clockwork.** You'll eat breakfast within one hour of waking up and then space your meals evenly throughout the day, three to five hours apart. This timing is critical to your success. On this eating schedule, you'll regulate your blood-sugar and insulin levels and your hunger hormones, reset and rev up your metabolism, and feel energized even while you're losing pounds and inches. If you eat the meals found in chapter 4 but there's a six-hour gap between lunch and dinner and just two hours between dinner and your evening snack, you aren't following the Cinch! plan. Meal timing is that important.

**Rule 2: Think, "Five Pieces Four Times a Day."** You'll prepare quick and easy meals that follow a unique "puzzle" constructed from five pieces:

1. Produce
2. A whole grain
3. Lean protein
4. Plant-based fat
5. Seasonings (which I collectively call SASS—Slimming And Satiating Seasonings)

Each meal contains all five pieces of the puzzle, and I'll tell you exactly how to assemble the parts. The precise puzzle configuration—strategic amounts of each of the five pieces—is a fundamental part of why this plan is so effective. That's because I calculated the ideal amounts from each food group needed to whittle away body fat while still allowing you to feel full, satisfied, energized, and nourished. And guess what? It's a lot of food! I'm happy to tell you that, unlike many weight-loss plans, my approach isn't about starving, restricting, or depriving yourself. It's all about giving your body precisely what it needs to get to your ideal weight and feel absolutely amazing every step of the way. What I especially love about this plan is that once the puzzle becomes second nature—and it will by the end of week one—you can put it into action no matter where you are: at a restaurant, on a cruise, or in your own kitchen. The puzzle principle will become your own personal blueprint for how to construct every meal with confidence, so you can stay on track, reach your goals, and relish your newfound sovereignty over excess pounds and an unhealthy relationship with food.

Rule 3: **Make Flavor Your Focus.** The fifth piece of the puzzle, SASS—Slimming And Satiating Seasonings—gives the "sizzle" to this plan. You'll doctor up every meal with one or more of the following five delicious additions:

1. Vinegar
2. Citrus juice or zest
3. Hot peppers
4. Tea
5. Herbs and spices

As a group these seasonings not only add layers of flavors but are the power of this plan, since exciting studies have found that each one brings the heat to fire up your fat-burning engine. They're also rich in antiaging, health-promoting antioxidants, which fascinating new research has linked to lower body-fat levels, even without dieting.

I've never believed that losing weight means sacrificing the flavor and enjoyment of food. On the Cinch! plan, I'll take you on a flavor journey. Along the way, you'll discover that you don't need butter, sugar, and salt to create delectable, satisfying meals. You can start your day with a Chocolate Pear Ginger Smoothie or Berry Almond French Toast. For lunch you can enjoy Black Bean Tacos with Cilantro-Jalapeño Guacamole, and

Green-Tea Chicken with Avocado Corn Salad. Dinner options include a Salmon Ginger Rice Bowl, and Turkey and Wild Rice Stuffed Peppers. Snacks are on the plan, too! You can indulge in an afternoon Pineapple Almond Peppercorn Parfait or a Vanilla Almond Frozen Banana. And here's the surprise: Cinch! makes a daily dark-chocolate escape your mandatory fifth meal, to be enjoyed whenever you like! Yes—*mandatory* chocolate!

Cinch! offers a wonderful variety of meals—even pasta! Egg- and cheese-based entrées are options, too, and there is a choice of all-natural, vegan meals made with beans and lentils. I created one hundred precise meals for you that follow the puzzle principle, but which meals you choose are up to you. Just select what you're in the mood for, make the meal as stated, and enjoy! If you're a creative cook, I also include a chapter that explains exactly how to use the puzzle principle to craft your own original Cinch! creations. And I tell you how to make take-along packs so you're never without a meal or snack and you can adhere to the meal timing to maximize your results.

> 24 25 26 27 28 29 30
>
> After years of struggling, I changed my relationship with food.
>
> JESS, AGE 30

All of the Cinch! meals in chapter 4 are terrifically simple, requiring minimal prep and cooking time. Even better, the plan offers delicious combinations you might never have considered, like serving spiced berries alongside your morning omelet or perking up your popcorn snack with Italian herbs, Parmesan, and cranberries. You'll see that your palate will welcome new tastes, and you'll soon have new favorite foods and recipes.

## the 5-day *fast forward*

The 5-Day Fast Forward is an über-streamlined clean-eating plan. Four simple, tasty meals each day made from just five extraordinary foods: spinach, almonds, raspberries, eggs, and yogurt (or vegan-friendly alternatives). I handpicked this short list because these five foods share three important characteristics: (1) each is filling, which means you won't be starving even though you're limiting your diet; (2) each contains natural detoxifying and health-protecting nutrients, so you'll be rejuvenating your body while you're losing weight; and (3) each has been shown in published research to specifically support weight loss.

Using these five superfoods in various combinations, I created four daily delicious meals. On the 5-Day Fast Forward plan, you repeat these same four meals every day for five days. The plan is ultrasimple, easy to follow, and repetitive. Just head to the market, load your cart with the items on the grocery list on page 37, and you have everything you need to move into action. These five days give your body, mind, and taste buds a fresh start and help you shed up to eight pounds. Keeping it simple gives your body a chance to reset itself and cleans your palate for the exciting plan to follow.

## is the 5-day *fast forward* plan for you?

In weight loss, as in life, there's no "one size fits all." Some people feel more confident and achieve better results with more structure, fewer choices, and lots of repetition. Others find those very things limiting or boring or even a bit scary. In my private practice, about half of my clients request a Fast Forward plan. When their choices are limited and the big decisions are left up to me and not them, they feel a sense of confidence and control. For this bunch, a clear-cut start feels manageable and trouble-free rather than overwhelming. Their attitude is: "Five days, no problem. Can I do it longer?" For the other half of my clients, a strict plan with a narrow list of foods triggers a feeling of rebellion. They begin to focus on all the foods they can't have, even if they love the foods on the strict plan. They tend to feel confined and may even quit before the end of day one or rebound overeat. To figure out on which side of the fence your feelings lie, take the following quiz. Remember that the Fast Forward plan is about getting a quick start on your weight-loss goal; you will move directly from the 5-Day Fast Forward into the full twenty-five-day program, where your food choices expand while you continue to lose weight.

## to *fast forward* or not: that is the question!

Please answer yes or no to each of the following questions:

Do you get excited when you learn about new ways to lose weight fast?   ☐ **yes**   ☐ **no**

Do your feelings of confidence and motivation soar when you follow a limited eating plan?   ☐ **yes**   ☐ **no**

Do you find it easier to stick to a plan if you know exactly what to eat and how much?   ☐ **yes**   ☐ **no**

Do your cravings dwindle once you get the "junk" out of your diet?   ☐ **yes**   ☐ **no**

Do you get frustrated when you have to figure out what to make for dinner?   ☐ **yes**   ☐ **no**

Do you tend to look forward to meals that include the same featured foods?   ☐ **yes**   ☐ **no**

If you answered yes to three or more of these questions, then the 5-Day Fast Forward is for you! However, even if you had more "no" answers than "yes" answers, I want you to carefully read the detailed plan in chapter 2 before you decide. You know yourself better than anyone else, so review the plan and listen to your gut instinct. If the idea of a stricter start isn't for you, then joyfully begin the amazing and effective Cinch! core program, which you will follow for the full thirty days. If you choose to start with the Fast Forward, you'll follow that plan for five days and the Cinch! core program for twenty-five days.

## the power of structure

As you can see, both Cinch! plans are precisely designed. This structure provides a powerful punch. Structure tells you what to do, but it also allows you to free your mind so you can explore your emotional connections to food. You learn the most about yourself when you let go of using food as a fix for boredom or stress and break your destructive habits and routines. Let's say you tend to eat simply because others around you are eating; when you are following this plan rather than mindlessly following the crowd, a lot of new thoughts and feelings will surface. To help you sort them out, I include a 5-Day Food Diary as an essential part of the Cinch! plan. It's a way for you to track not only what, how much, and when you're eating, but also how you're feeling—both physically and emotionally.

> 24 25 26 27 28 29 30
>
> I've done very extreme programs in the past. This is something I can live with for life.
>
> CHRIS, AGE 54

Whether you start with the Fast Forward plan or the Cinch! core plan, fill in the diary starting from day one. The brief "homework" assignments contained in the diary will begin to untangle the *whys* of your eating—why you have been eating too much or making poor food choices—along with your social and emotional connections to food. Answering these questions thoroughly and truthfully will form the real groundwork for change.

## reconnect with your body

On the Cinch! plan, I want you to feel mild to moderate hunger about four times a day. Hunger is a normal physical sensation that acts as a bridge between your body and mind so they can work together to keep you in balance. When you were an infant, all your food decisions were guided completely by your body. You cried when you needed food and

# MY STORY

## Selena Shepps, age 24  |  Pounds lost: 10

# I Transformed My Middle!

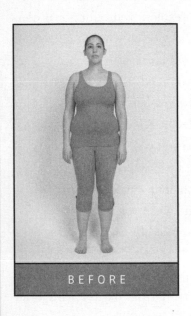

BEFORE

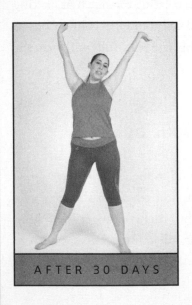

AFTER 30 DAYS

Cinch! is my hero! I love everything about it and it is hands down the simplest, most nourishing way to eat and lose weight.

I work in the music industry, managing artist websites. I also have my own skincare business and I'm on the board of the nonprofit organization Women in Music. I'm self-motivated and passionate about my career, but I wasn't taking care of my body. I've been eating fast food all my life and beverages were a major challenge for me. I had a huge problem saying no to soda! Out of habit, I snacked when I wasn't hungry and I added way too much salt to my food.

I alternated my unhealthy habits with just about every diet out there, but they always left me tired, hungry, unsatisfied, moody, anxious, and disappointed. I would lose weight and then be stuck, because as soon as I would alter one step, the weight was back and my jeans were tight again.

On Cinch!, my body and mind improved after the first day and in less than a week the "puzzle" became second nature. I went on autopilot. It's soooo easy. The puzzle strategy is pure genius. I no longer feel sick after eating, have a steady flow of energy, and I never feel like I'm limiting myself. The four meals a day are easy to prepare, and leave me with the perfect level of fullness. I can really feel the lifestyle change.

Cinch! also helped me forget about

sugary beverages and junk food. What else can you ask for? It's like winning the lotto.

One of my favorite things about Cinch! is that I started making my own meals instead of grabbing whatever was available. I've wanted to learn how to cook for a while. Now I don't need a cooking class. I have the basics down and I can make one hundred meals! All of the meals are clear and simple, and I have the ability to mix them up anytime just by using a little creativity or substitutions. It's awesome!

After thirty days I felt like I've been eating this way forever because everything is so natural. In fact my body is so used to my Cinch! plan that I think it would revolt against me if I ever changed back to my bad eating habits. Now I know that I'm capable of taking care of my body. And I certainly love to see those numbers go down on the scale! It's exhilarating! I'll never have to Photoshop a picture again or make a friend delete a photo because it's a "bad angle." I have more to lose but with Cinch! I'm certain I will be able to do it. I'm not thinking about food, calories, or sugary beverages. I'm only thinking about myself and the lifestyle I want. And I'm making it happen!

I think my new eating confidence is transferring over to my everyday tasks. I had a big project at work and I would normally have asked co-workers for help, but I had enough confidence to give it a shot myself. I simply looked at the situation, figured out what I had to do, and did it. It's just like Cinch! Figure out the puzzle, get the ingredients, commit, and repeat!

stopped nursing when your body told your brain that you'd had enough. You ate small, frequent "meals" and were completely unaware of any eating motivation other than wanting to feel happy and good.

We don't feel happy and good when we're starving—that's why babies cry when their bodies tell them they need food—or when we're overly full or stuffed. Overeating disrupts your circulation by diverting blood away from your brain, muscles, and vital organs and toward your digestive system. Less oxygen and fewer nutrients are available to your body, and you feel sluggish and fatigued. Babies rarely feel this way, because they instinctively eat in a way that is designed to make them feel nourished, satisfied, and content. It's the "Goldilocks" outcome: not too much, not too little, just right. Through Cinch! you'll reconnect with the internal eating guide you were born with and learn to trust and honor it again.

## the cinch! beverages

Cinch! is all about giving your body the most nutritious, clean, natural options, for both foods and beverages. The beverage rules that follow will guide you. They apply to both the Fast Forward and core Cinch! plan.

Cinch! beverage options:

- Water, iced or hot; minimum of eight cups, maximum of two and a half liters (ten cups) per day.
- All-natural, calorie-free seltzer. The only ingredients you should see on the can or bottle are carbonated water and natural flavoring. Count seltzer toward your total water intake.
- All-natural, calorie-free, flavored flat water (no bubbles). The only ingredients you should see are water and natural flavoring. Count flat water toward your total water intake.
- Freshly brewed iced or hot black, oolong, green, white, red, or herbal tea, unsweetened; maximum of five cups per day.

- Bottled unsweetened brewed iced tea, flat or sparkling. Count toward your total tea intake.
- Coffee; limit of one cup (eight ounces) per day, with maximum of one-quarter cup organic skim or organic soy milk, no artificial sweeteners; add one teaspoon or one packet raw sugar if desired, and flavor with spices such as cinnamon, nutmeg, or cloves. Soy milks labeled vanilla or plain generally have about the equivalent of two cubes of sugar added per cup. If you use these flavors, as opposed to unsweetened soy milk, don't add the packet of raw sugar. (If you're not a coffee drinker, you can skip this, but you don't get to add an additional cup of tea to compensate.)
- Zesty Cinnamon Basil Berry Tea, maximum of one recipe per day:

## Zesty Cinnamon Basil Berry Tea

1 bag green tea
¼ cup 100 percent Concord grape juice
1 cinnamon stick
¼ teaspoon freshly grated orange or tangerine zest (use organic fruit to avoid pesticide residue)
3 sweet basil leaves, torn
Unflavored all-natural seltzer (optional)

1. In a large mug, add tea bag to 6 ounces boiling water.
2. Use cinnamon stick to stir in the juice and zest. Leave cinnamon stick in mug.
3. Add basil and steep, covered, for five minutes.
4. Remove tea bag but leave all other ingredients and enjoy.

Optional cold beverage version: chill tea, transfer to a tumbler, and mix with ½ cup effervescent all-natural seltzer. The longer the tea sits in the refrigerator, the more it becomes infused with flavor. You can even chill it overnight, but for freshness, be sure to drink or discard within twenty-four hours.

This beautifully hued beverage blends the subtle flavors of green tea, berry (grapes are—surprise!—a member of the berry family), basil, cinnamon, and orange zest. Plus, it's loaded with antiaging disease fighters.

Concord grapes are bursting with antioxidants called polyphenols, particularly a subgroup called flavonoids. The natural pigment that gives Concord grapes their vibrant tint is rich in antioxidants that aren't found in red, green, white, or yellow/orange produce, and studies show that 88 percent of Americans fall short on produce from this color family, more than any other group.

The antioxidants in green tea, also flavonoids, are protective against a number of diseases. Studies show that compared to people who drink less than one cup of green tea per day, those who sip at least five cups have a significantly lower risk of death from all causes, specifically from heart disease, the nation's number one killer of men and women. Plus, substances in green tea known as catechins trigger weight loss.

I have added cinnamon not only for its lovely aroma and flavor but also because this amazing spice has consistently been shown to slow the rate at which the stomach empties after a meal, reducing the postmeal rise in blood sugar and making you feel fuller longer. Plus, cinnamon is rich in antioxidants—you'll find as substantial a dose in 1 teaspoon of cinnamon as you will in a half cup of blueberries.

Basil, a member of the mint family, is commonly used in Thailand, India, and Turkey as a medicinal herb to improve digestion and promote relaxation. Antioxidants in basil protect your cells from the damage caused by stress and inflammation and promote healing. Gently tearing the leaves will release the essential oils, which have been shown to possess anticancer, antiviral, and antimicrobial properties. To learn about why I included citrus zest, see page 77 in chapter 3 (hint: I refer to zest as one of nature's fat burners and another potent immune booster).

## say no to soda

It won't surprise you to learn that soda is not part of the Cinch! plan. In my experience, parting ways with soft drinks for good is one of the most important steps you can take for your health and waistline. Sweetened drinks are the number one source of sugar in the American diet, and the consumption of sugary drinks has jumped by 70 percent since 1970. Americans today average fifty gallons of soda and other sweetened beverages each year.

This is an enormous problem because, as research shows, liquids are less satisfying than solid food. Beverages simply don't appear to register with our appetite controls. In a four-week study at Purdue University, volunteers were provided 450 calories per day as either soda or jelly beans; beyond that, they were allowed to eat whatever they wanted. In the end, the soda group consumed 17 percent more total calories than the jelly-bean group, and only the soda group gained weight. The lesson, of course, is not that jelly beans are good for weight control but that liquid calories will put you on the fast track to an expanded waistline. One can of sweetened soda a day can turn into fifteen pounds of body fat a year!

Soda not only is bad for your waistline but also can sabotage your health. Statistically, people who consume more sugar tend to eat more calories and fewer nutrients because empty-calorie foods and drinks such as soda tend to squeeze out nutrient-rich choices whose calories are bundled with vitamins, minerals, fiber, and antioxidants (e.g., soda instead of fresh fruit).

Plus, a higher intake of added sugar is tied to nearly every chronic disease, including type 2 diabetes, heart disease, high blood pressure, certain cancers, even Alzheimer's. A twenty-ounce bottle of cola packs 250 calories from a whopping sixty-eight grams of sugar—that's seventeen teaspoons' worth—far exceeding the American Heart Association's maximum daily recommended cap of six teaspoons of added sugar for women and nine teaspoons for men.

Soda has also been tied to a higher risk of nonalcoholic fatty liver disease (NAFLD) and kidney disease. An Israeli study published in the *Journal of Hepatology* found that the more soft drinks the subjects consumed, the more likely they were to have NAFLD. Scientists from the Loyola University Health System found that women who drink two or more cans of regular soda pop per day are nearly twice as likely to show early signs of kidney disease. Those who reported drinking two or more sodas in the twenty-four hours before the study were 1.86 times more likely to have albuminuria, an excess amount of a protein in urine, often symptomatic of kidney damage.

> 24  25  26  27  28  29  30
>
> I love that all the meals are customized. Since I'm a vegetarian, it always takes so much effort to custom-ize many diet plans. But you've already done that for me!
>
> AMY, AGE 28

## diet soda is out, too!

Most people assume diet soda is okay, even encouraged, on a diet. (After all, it *is* called "diet" soda.) But—brace yourself, diet-drink lovers—artificial sweeteners aren't part of the Cinch! plan. Why not? The short answer: I don't believe artificial sweeteners help you lose weight, I don't think they're good for your health, and I don't believe they belong in our food supply.

I didn't always feel this way. As a health professional with degrees in science, I've been trained to think about things like odds ratios, which are basically risk comparisons, or the chances that a given outcome will occur based on various risk factors. For example, there are many behaviors linked to cancer, but the chances, or "odds," of being diagnosed with cancer are much higher for a twenty-year smoker than for, say, a person who has had a few X-rays. But that doesn't really mean X-rays are safe; it just means they aren't as risky.

When it comes to artificial sweeteners, the government has set an Acceptable Daily Intake, or ADI—the level of a substance that a person can safely consume every day over a lifetime without the risk of developing serious side effects. ADI is determined by toxicity studies, mostly in animals. I used to look at those numbers and think, "Okay, a person would have to consume an awful lot of aspartame—about twenty cans of diet cola per day—to reach the ADI," but my philosophy has shifted. Over the years, I began to combine my training in statistics and science with intuition and experience, and I started asking larger questions, such as: How did our culture even get to a place where we have created artificial sugar that requires toxicology tests?

Conflicting studies about the safety of artificial sweeteners, combined with complaints from clients of mine whose headaches, dizziness, and mood changes vanished after they purged the fake stuff from their diets, led me to add artificial sweeteners to my list of substances that I don't feel good about.

Finally, over the decades in which fake sugars have been available, obesity rates have continued to skyrocket, and both animal and human studies tie these substances to weight gain rather than weight loss. A Purdue University study published in *Behavioral Neuroscience* found that rats fed yogurt sweetened with zero-calorie saccharin later consumed more calories, gained more weight, and packed on more body fat than did rats fed sugar-sweetened yogurt. Other animal studies indicate that artificial sweeteners may throw off the body's natural ability to regulate calories.

Statistically, the human risk of obesity actually increases with each daily serving of diet soda, even more so than it does for regular soda drinkers! One study found that for people who drank one to two cans of diet soda a day, the risk of becoming overweight or obese was 54.5 percent, compared with 32.8 percent for people drinking the same amount of sugar-sweetened soda.

I also became much more aware of the circle of sustainability—how the effects of food production and what we eat impact the environment and the integrity of our entire food system. That's another mark against artificial sweeteners. European research has found that artificial sweeteners don't get removed in wastewater treatment. One study detected acesulfame, cyclamate, saccharin, and sucralose in waters from two German sewage-treatment plants. This indicated that the treatments failed to cleanse the sweeteners from wastewater, allowing them to continue downstream and remain present in drinking water. Scientists say that a sugarlike chemical lingering in the environment could potentially impact how various organisms feed, interfere with plant photosynthesis, and lead to algae problems.

Bottom line: artificial sweeteners are, well, *artificial*. They don't add nutritional value to your food, and they may have unwanted side effects for both you and the environment.

I know you may feel that it is hard to give them up, especially if you've been dependent on them for years for that satisfying taste of sweetness; but, honestly, it's easy to avoid them. You'll be surprised how quickly your taste buds adjust. I had one client who used to put six to eight packets of artificial sweetener in her coffee every morning. Before long, she was perfectly happy with one packet of raw sugar and a dash of cinnamon.

## what about alcohol?

I haven't included an "alcohol allowance" on this plan because alcohol doesn't contribute to weight loss, it isn't essential for health, and research shows that even moderate drinking—one drink a day—can increase the risk of breast cancer. In chapter 10, I give you guidelines for enjoying alcohol *after* you reach your goal weight. If you really miss alcohol, just remember that once you've reached your goal weight, you can have an occasional drink of alcohol, and I'll tell you how to do that without gaining weight. Until then, you'll be enjoying delightful nonalcoholic beverages while slimming to a spectacular new you!

## ready, set, go!

Just thirty days from today you'll be slimmer—losing pounds and inches. Just as important, you also will have mastered a new way of eating that optimizes your health, gives you boundless energy, is deliciously satisfying, and is easy to follow anytime, anyplace. Cinch! is the way you've always wanted to eat but never knew how.

In chapter 2, I introduce you to the 5-Day, 5-Food Fast Forward plan. Even if you think you want to opt out of the Fast Forward and are eager to start the core Cinch! plan, I encourage you to read chapter 2. It includes an in-depth look at the five slimming superfoods—spinach, almonds, raspberries, eggs, yogurt, and vegan alternatives—that not only give you a super start but are some of the powerhouse foods featured throughout the plan.

Let's get started and lose some weight!

# 2

`24 25 26 27 28 29 30 31 32 33`

# the 5-day,
# 5-food fast forward

You've taken the quiz in chapter 1 (on page 16) and decided that the 5-Day Fast Forward is right up your alley. I'm sure you're excited to dive right in, but first I want to tell you about three important goals you'll accomplish over the next five days:

**1. You'll lose weight—up to eight pounds.** Even within the first forty-eight hours you'll begin to feel lighter, more energized, and less bloated. And seeing a quick drop on the scale and a loosening of your clothes will empower you to gear up for the full twenty-five-day Cinch! core to follow.

**2. You'll gain confidence.** Yup, the Fast Forward plan is strict, but that's the point: the rigor of the plan is its power. Being able to follow such a specific plan will give you as much confidence as the weight loss itself. Nothing feels better than meeting a challenging goal. Completing the 5-Day, 5-Food Fast Forward will give you the self-assurance that you can finish the much more open twenty-five day Cinch! core and transition to a pattern of healthful eating that you can sustain for life.

**3. You'll reconnect with your body.** This week, I want you to feel mild to moderate hunger about four times a day. An appropriate pattern of hunger and fullness is one of the important keys to losing weight and keeping it off, and you'll be back in sync with that pattern within the next few days.

NOTE: As easy as it is, I don't want you to follow this plan for more than five days. Five days is all you need to jump-start your body, and this plan is too limited in variety to meet your body's diverse nutrient needs over the long term.

## get ready to say good-bye to your spanx!

On page 37, you'll find the complete grocery list for the plan. I recommend shopping one day before you start the program and purchasing all of the foods at once so that everything is in place to prepare your meals and eat on schedule. Staying away from the supermarket can also help you avoid temptation. I also recommend that you explain your mission to everyone who lives in your household so that they can offer encouragement and support. The last thing you want is your spouse making dinner reservations or bringing home a piping hot pizza on day three of your Fast Forward. Remind your partner about a time when he or she needed your help, something that was important—like going for a promotion or new job or starting a new workout program or hobby. Say something like, "Remember when you needed my help with [fill in the blank]? Well, this

> I was happy with every single meal I had today and felt great!
> KARLA, AGE 34

is just as important to me. It's like the beginning of a new chapter in my life, so please don't tempt me to get off track. I need you to be my cheer-leader as much as you can." Finally, share your Fast Forward plans with close friends. Maybe one of them will even want to join you!

## the five *fast forward* foods

You'll notice that I recommend shopping for some organic options here. If I could eat 100 percent organic I would, but that's not practical due to the extra cost. That's why I've singled out certain foods in particular. For those where I note organic, I strongly feel that the exceptional qual-ity, nutritional value, and safety of organic versus conventional versions are worth the extra cost. If that's a deal breaker, I'd prefer to see you buy conventional and follow the plan rather than chuck the whole thing. As a nutritionist, my goals are to help you lose weight while ensuring the best possible nutritional status and health. I do believe that some organic foods provide an edge nutritionally and health-wise, but will you still achieve weight-loss results with conventional versions? Yes. Bottom line: select organic options when noted if they're available and if your food budget allows. If not, an all-natural version is the next best thing. (See page 205 for more information on how to save on organic foods.)

- Spinach
- Raspberries
- Almonds
- Organic eggs[*]
- Nonfat (0 percent) plain organic yogurt[**]

---

[*] Vegetarians and vegans substitute organic unflavored extra-firm tofu.
[**] Vegans and non-dairy eaters substitute organic plain soy yogurt or plain coconut-milk yogurt.

## sip yourself slimmer

Can green tea help you lose weight? It appears so. According to research in the *Journal of Nutrition,* antioxidants in green tea called catechins helped exercisers shed more fat. In the twelve-week study, a group that worked out at a moderate intensity three hours a week and daily consumed a green tea drink containing 625 mg of catechins, the amount in about six cups of green tea, lost twice as much weight as, and significantly more belly fat than, a group that performed the same workout regimen but drank a catechin-free beverage.

Green tea's magic is still a mystery, but scientists believe catechins may trigger a preference for burning fat instead of carbohydrates.

Grocery Guidelines

- Spinach can be fresh or frozen.
- Raspberries can be fresh or frozen.
- Almonds can be sliced or slivered, plus you will eat 2 tablespoons of almond butter each day.
- Eggs can include one large whole organic egg, whites from three large fresh organic eggs, ¼ cup organic liquid egg whites, or ½ cup organic extra-firm tofu.

*Fast Forward* Seasonings

- Vinegar, any type, with 0 mg sodium and no more than 15 calories per tablespoon. Limit to 6 tablespoons per day.
- Citrus juice or wedges—maximum ¼ cup 100 percent citrus juice per day, which can include any type, from lemon or lime to blood orange, tangerine, or pink grapefruit.
- Garlic—fresh, roasted, or minced and jarred in water. No limit.

- Hot peppers, fresh or dried, such as jalapeño, serrano, or Thai chili peppers. Limit to three whole peppers per day.
- Fresh or dried salt-free herbs and spices of any kind. No limit.

### *Fast Forward* Beverages

- Water, iced or hot; minimum of eight cups, maximum of two and a half liters (ten cups), per day.
- All-natural, calorie-free seltzer. The only ingredients you should see on the can or bottle are carbonated water and natural flavoring. Count seltzer toward your total water intake.
- All-natural, calorie-free, flavored flat water (no bubbles). The only ingredients you should see are water and natural flavoring. Count flat water toward your total water intake.
- Freshly brewed iced or hot black, oolong, green, white, red, or herbal tea, unsweetened; maximum of five cups per day.
- Bottled unsweetened brewed iced tea, flat or sparkling. Count toward your total tea intake.
- Coffee; limit of one cup (eight ounces) per day, with maximum of one-quarter cup organic skim or organic soy milk, no artificial sweeteners; add one teaspoon or one packet raw sugar if desired, and flavor with spices such as cinnamon, nutmeg, or cloves. Soy milks labeled vanilla or plain generally have about the equivalent of two cubes of sugar added per cup. If you use these flavors, as opposed to unsweetened soy milk, don't add the packet of raw sugar. (If you're not a coffee drinker, you can skip this, but you don't get to add an additional cup of tea to compensate.)
- Zesty Cinnamon Basil Berry Tea, maximum of one recipe per day. (See page 21 for the recipe.)

# *fast forward* meals

Here are your meals, along with sample times that you might eat depending on your daily schedule. Of course, if you work a swing shift or a night shift, your mealtimes will be entirely different, but they should reflect the same schedule of eating within an hour of waking up and then going no shorter than three hours and no longer than five hours between meals.

## Scramble (8:00 A.M.)

1 cup spinach, fresh, or frozen and thawed

¼ cup organic egg whites, 1 whole organic egg, or whites from 3 large organic eggs, ¼ cup organic liquid egg whites, (or ⅕ of a 14-oz package organic extra-firm tofu)

Approved seasonings

1 cup raspberries, fresh or frozen

2 tablespoons almonds, sliced or slivered

Mix fresh or thawed frozen spinach with egg or tofu, add seasonings of your choice, and scramble in pan using extra-virgin olive oil cooking spray. Serve with a side of raspberries, sprinkled with sliced or slivered almonds; 2 cups water; and, if desired, 1 cup other approved beverage.

SEASONING SUGGESTIONS: Add 1 teaspoon minced garlic and a dash of cracked black pepper or crushed red pepper to eggs or tofu, or use minced garlic with a dash of turmeric.

## Parfait (12:30 P.M.)

6 ounces nonfat (0 percent) plain organic yogurt (or plain organic soy or coconut-milk yogurt)

1 cup raspberries, fresh, or frozen and thawed

2 tablespoons almonds, sliced or slivered

Approved seasonings

Season the ingredients, and then layer them parfait-style. Serve with 2 cups water and, if desired, 1 cup other approved beverage.

SEASONING SUGGESTION: Lightly dust berries with cinnamon, nutmeg, cloves, or a mixture of all three, and add three or four freshly chopped mint leaves to the yogurt.

## yes, you do need eight cups of water a day!

Water has been a typical component of weight-loss plans for decades, and I include a minimum of eight cups a day on Cinch! However, this age-old recommendation has come under fire in the media recently, with headlines such as "Idea All Wet: You Don't Need 8 Glasses of Water a Day."

The backlash started after a few researchers wrote an editorial in a scientific journal concluding that there is "no medical evidence" that we need eight glasses a day.

Well, I beg to differ. Water is the single most important nutrient. You can survive six weeks without food but only seven days without water. About 60 to 70 percent of the human body is made of water. Water is required for every single bodily process, and every minute of every day you continuously lose water from your body—through your skin (to help regulate your body temperature) and when you breathe (every time you exhale). Water vapor is what interacts with cold air to allow you to "see your breath" on a chilly night, and holding a mirror up to someone's nose or mouth when they're unconscious is a common way to check for breathing, because water vapor will mist the mirror.

About 20 percent of our daily water needs are generally met by food (even more if you eat several servings of water-filled fresh produce), and the rest comes from beverages, whether water itself or other fluids.

According to the Institute of Medicine (IOM), women aged nineteen and up need 2.7 liters of total fluid per day (over eleven cups) and men need 3.7 liters (over fifteen cups). Studies tell us that most Americans drink about 2 liters of

## Salad (5:30 P.M.)

2 cups fresh spinach
1 cup raspberries, fresh, or frozen and thawed
2 tablespoons almonds, sliced or slivered
1 large organic egg or whites from 3 large fresh organic eggs, hard-boiled (or ⅓ of a 14-oz package extra-firm organic tofu, cubed or crumbled)
Approved seasonings

Season spinach, toss with berries, almonds, and egg or tofu, and add further seasoning of choice. Serve with 2 cups water and, if desired, 1 cup other approved beverage.

total beverages per day, but less than a quarter of that amount comes from water. Technically, nonwater drinks like soda, lemonade, and sweet tea do "count" toward your fluid needs, even if they contain caffeine, as long as you're consistent. But of course those drinks can also provide empty calories (calories that aren't bundled with valuable nutrients) and can contribute to weight gain. To meet your body's fluid needs and "put back" what you're losing, pure water is best. Even if 20 percent of your fluids come from food, that still leaves eight to twelve cups based on the IOM's guidelines.

According to a study in the *American Journal of Clinical Nutrition,* people who get a good part of their daily liquids from plain water rather than other beverages have healthier diets overall. Using data from a national health survey of more than twelve thousand Americans, researchers found that people who drank more plain water tended to eat more fiber, less sugar, and fewer high-calorie foods.

Will drinking water burn extra calories? There's little research on the topic, but a German study showed that a sixteen-ounce dose of water increased metabolic rate by 30 percent within ten minutes, peaking thirty to forty minutes after consumption. The effect was sustained for more than an hour. The authors concluded that drinking two liters of water a day could burn up to 95 extra calories.

If you're like most people, you may not need to drink more; you just need to drink differently. That means trading in regular or diet soda for the "approved beverages" on my list. Once you get into the routine, an ice-cold glass of H₂O or a mug of green tea will become your go-to drink in no time.

---

SEASONING SUGGESTION: Toss spinach with 2 tablespoons balsamic vinegar and 1 tablespoon freshly squeezed citrus juice, such as tangerine or blood orange. Top with berries, almonds, and egg or tofu, and garnish salad with freshly grated pepper or a dusting of cracked black pepper.

## Smoothie (10:00 P.M.)

6 ounces nonfat (0 percent) plain organic yogurt
(or plain organic soy yogurt or coconut-milk yogurt)
1 cup raspberries, fresh, or frozen and thawed

2 tablespoons natural almond butter
Small handful ice
Approved seasonings

Whip yogurt, raspberries, almond butter, ice, and seasonings, if desired, in blender until smooth. Serve with 2 cups water and, if desired, 1 cup other approved beverage.

SEASONING SUGGESTION: Add ½ to 1 teaspoon freshly grated ginger or ½ teaspoon cinnamon to smoothie.

## *fast forward* rules

Keeping it simple is the key to this plan. Here is all you have to do each day:

- Eat your first meal within one hour of waking up.
- Eat one of each meal per day, in any order you like, spacing your meals evenly, three to five hours apart.
- Use only the foods, beverages, and seasonings listed.

## why i chose the five *fast forward* foods

Over the next five days, you'll become quite familiar with these five superstar foods (or their vegan-friendly alternatives), and each one remains an important foundation throughout the entire thirty-day plan. These foods will help you lose weight and support your body with the spectacular nutrients they contain, and I'll teach you how to shop for the tastiest varieties.

Fact ───────────────────────────────

Oleic acid, found in "good" fats such as almonds and extra-virgin olive oil, triggers your small intestine to produce oleoylethanolamide, a compound that curbs hunger pangs, according to a recent study from the University of California at Irvine. One of the best sources of oleic acid? Almonds!

# *fast forward* grocery list

Here's exactly what you'll need to buy to make five days' worth of Fast Forward meals:

**Spinach**—15 cups total:
15 cups loose, fresh; or
7 clamshells fresh; or
5 10-ounce bags frozen

**Raspberries**—20 cups total:
20 half-pint containers fresh or
10 10-ounce bags frozen

**Almonds**—30 tablespoons total, sliced or slivered, plus 10 tablespoons almond butter:
4 cups bulk sliced or slivered or
2 6-ounce bags sliced or slivered almonds and
1 jar natural almond butter

**Organic eggs**—10 whole, 30 whole whites, or 5 cups liquid egg whites total:
1 carton whole eggs or
3 cartons for whole whites or
3 16-ounce containers liquid egg whites

**Yogurt**—60 ounces total:
10 6-ounce containers or
2 32-ounce tubs

**Tofu** (to replace eggs if desired)—
5 cups (about 42 ounces) total:
3 14-ounce packages

You can also purchase the optional but encouraged SASS ingredients and approved beverages. You may want to add these items to your grocery list:

1 can extra-virgin olive oil cooking spray

1 bottle balsamic vinegar

1 bag fresh citrus such as clementines or tangerines

1 bulb garlic or 1 jar minced garlic in water

Fresh hot peppers such as jalapeños or Thai chili peppers

Fresh ginger

1 bunch fresh mint

1 prefilled grinder peppercorn

1 prefilled grinder Italian herbs such as Melissa's brand (www.melissas.com)

Turmeric

Crushed red pepper

Ground cinnamon and cinnamon sticks

Nutmeg

Cloves

1 bunch fresh basil

1 box green-tea bags

## spectacular spinach

Sure, spinach fills you up for very few calories—for the same calories you'd consume in a half cup of cooked brown rice (100 calories), you could eat twenty cups of spinach! But that's not the only reason these leafy greens help you stay slim.

It turns out, the antioxidants and other natural substances abundant in spinach may help ward off the metabolic processes that lead to obesity and heart disease. In a recent University of Florida study, published in the *Journal of Human Nutrition and Dietetics,* researchers analyzed the dietary patterns of fifty-four adults—half normal weight, half overweight-obese—over a three-day period and repeated the analysis eight weeks later. Although the two groups consumed about the same number of total calories, the normal-weight group ate about four times more leafy greens. They also had lower levels of inflammation—a known trigger of premature aging, obesity, heart disease, diabetes, and joint diseases. A new report revealed that 69 percent of Americans do not get the minimum recommended amount of green produce: three cups per week.

*Natural Detoxer: Vitamin A.* Vitamin A is required for normal functioning of the immune system. You need vitamin A to keep your immune system set at "ready to pounce." This critical vitamin helps form skin cells as well as the lining inside your nasal passages and digestive tract, which form barriers that keep viruses and bacteria out of your body. The stronger and healthier those barriers are, the lower your chances of getting sick if

---

**Fact**

One cup of spinach leaves, the size of a baseball, provides just 5 calories—twenty times fewer calories than a half cup of cooked brown rice or whole-wheat pasta. This superfood may be light on calories, but it's rich in over a dozen stress-fighting antioxidants that help your body recover faster from the wear and tear of a workout or a particularly trying day!

## why frozen is as good as fresh

Will you compromise your Fast Forward plan if you use frozen spinach and raspberries instead of fresh? Absolutely not!

In fact, produce on ice can be even more nutrient-packed than fresh. That's because the moment a fruit or veggie is picked, it starts to lose nutrients, whereas freezing slows down that loss. One study found that the vitamin C content of fresh broccoli plunged by 56 percent in one week's time but dropped just 10 percent over the course of a year when frozen at −4°F (−20°C). Also, freezing actually boosts the levels of disease-fighting, antiaging antioxidants and some minerals, such as potassium, which helps control blood pressure. (You can learn more about this amazing mineral on page 258.)

Though fresh greens are available year-round, for convenience I always keep some frozen on hand. Frozen means no washing or chopping required, and you can stock up in case you can't get to the grocery store or you live in a cold climate, without a year-round farmer's market. Although I try to stockpile berries when they're in season and freeze them for the winter months, store-bought frozen varieties are a terrific option. See page 45 for tips on freezing greens and berries.

You can buy private-label (store-brand), brand-name, or generic frozen produce. Just stick with U.S. Grade A, also known as Fancy. Grade A or Fancy on the label indicates that the produce was carefully selected for color and tenderness. Fancy varieties tend to be more flavorful, compared with Grade B, also called Extra Standard.

This second-level grade means the produce is slightly more mature, so it may taste less fresh. Grade C, known as Standard, is the lowest grade; it generally means the produce won't be consistent in color or flavor and can sometimes be stringy or tough. You'll generally see the grades or terms on the front side of a package, or they may appear inside a symbol that looks like a shield.

When you buy frozen, make sure you choose brands with zero additives. The only ingredient you should see listed is the fruit or vegetable itself.

Bottom line: You don't have to shop only the perimeter of the store or bust your food budget to load up on nutritious produce.

Fact ——————————————————————————
Some 85 percent of people with type 2 diabetes eat too much saturated fat, 92 percent
consume excess sodium, and less than 50 percent meet the minimum fruit and veggie
recommendation, a recent study found. You can take control. People who eat well,
exercise, don't smoke, don't drink excessively, and aren't overweight are 89 percent less
likely to develop diabetes.

you're exposed to germs. Vitamin A also plays a central role in the development of white blood cells, such as lymphocytes—a critical component of your body's immune response. One cup of spinach has nearly 400 percent of your daily vitamin A requirement.

*Health Bonus:* Studies show that eating just one more daily serving of green leafy vegetables than you were before you started this plan can lower your risk of heart disease by 11 percent and of type 2 diabetes by 9 percent. Also, research has linked a high intake of leafy green salads to a substantially lower risk of dying from any cause. Spinach is rich in folate, a mineral linked to lower risk of heart disease and stroke, and in antioxidants shown to prevent damage to artery walls, especially in the bends and curves that are most vulnerable to inflammation.

Fact ——————————————————————————
Research shows that folate-rich foods slash women's risk of colorectal cancer by about
50 percent at least. Spinach is one of the top sources of folic acid, along with asparagus,
broccoli, beans, and lentils.

*Stock Up:* When buying fresh spinach, look for bags, clamshell containers, or loose leaves that have a deep, vibrant green color with no signs of yellow or brown. Avoid buying spinach that looks wilted, bruised, or slimy—signs that the leaves are past their prime and will decay quickly. Store fresh spinach loosely packed in a sealable container in the refrigerator crisper, where it will keep fresh for about five days. Do not wash it before storing, because the moisture will cause spoilage. Don't store cooked spinach; it won't keep well. For tips on buying frozen spinach, check out the box on page 39.

## irresistible almonds

Almonds are among the most decadent foods around; they're also among the most researched when it comes to weight loss. A study published in the *International Journal of Obesity and Related Metabolic Disorders* found that a low-calorie, almond-enriched diet helped overweight people shed more pounds than a low-caloric diet higher in complex carbohydrates. Both groups of dieters ate the same number of calories and equivalent amounts of protein, but after six months, those on the almond-enriched diet lost more weight and had smaller waistlines, less body fat, and lower systolic blood pressure. In fact, almond eaters experienced a 62 percent greater reduction in their body weight, a 50 percent greater loss in waist circumference, and a 56 percent greater loss of body fat.

Previous studies have found that eating nuts regularly reduces the risk of weight gain and obesity. A twenty-eight-month Spanish study involving more than eight thousand men and women found that those who ate nuts, including almonds, at least two times per week were 31 percent less likely to gain weight than people who never or rarely ate nuts. Recent research also has found that the monounsaturated fat in almonds is more satisfying than saturated fat, even at the same calorie level. A study from the University of Texas Southwestern Medical Center reported that the

> It really helps to be open about this and ask friends for support. Pretty much every one of my close friends and co-workers knows what I'm doing, so I've ensured that no one's going to pressure me to deviate from this plan. And it helps to talk about it and have that external support.
> AMY, AGE 28

Fact ───────────────────────────────

The number of households who grew their own fruits, veggies, and herbs in 2009 was 19 percent higher than in 2008.

saturated fat from butter, cheese, milk, and beef may signal the body's cells to ignore appetite-suppressing signals but that the healthy monounsaturated fat found in almonds does not.

*Natural Detoxer: Magnesium.* Magnesium triggers veins and arteries to relax, which reduces blood pressure and improves the flow of blood, oxygen, and nutrients throughout the body. Magnesium also is required for the production of DNA and protein in your body and plays a structural role in bones, cell membranes, and chromosomes. One ounce of almonds provides 20 percent of the magnesium you need each day.

*Health Bonus:* Almonds are bursting with minerals, B vitamins, and vitamin E, one of the body's key antioxidants, plus fiber and protein. Numerous studies have also shown that almonds help slash "bad" LDL cholesterol and lower blood pressure to lower the risk of heart disease.

Fact ————————————————————————————
More than 97 percent of women over age nineteen lack adequate intakes of vitamin E, an antioxidant that protects our cells from the effects of free radicals. Almonds are one of the best sources of vitamin E.

*Stock Up:* I'm a fan of almonds in any form, but for the Fast Forward, I decided to use sliced or slivered almonds and almond butter because they work best in my recipes. At the market, you'll find several brands of sliced or slivered almonds sold in bags, and they're often stocked in the bulk section. Any brand is fine; just make sure they're unsalted. To save money and eliminate additives when buying almond butter, look for grind-your-own machines at the supermarket or jars of all-natural brands with no added fats or sugars, such as Artisana or Mara Natha. The jar should contain just one ingredient: almonds.

## berries, beautiful berries

Fewer than 30 percent of adults eat the recommended two servings of fruit a day, and this void could be a culprit in the creeping obesity rate. Studies suggest that people who load up on fruits are even more likely to have lower body weight than frequent vegetable eaters. Raspberries in particular are a hidden treasure of nutrients tied to weight loss and good health.

Fact ──────────────────────────────────────────────────

At least 20 percent of the population qualifies as obese in forty-nine states and Washington, D.C. (Colorado is the lone standout.) Since 1988, the percentage of Americans who aren't overweight, exercise at least twelve times a month, don't smoke, and eat five or more servings of fruits and veggies per day has dropped from 15 percent to 8 percent. We can reverse this trend!

────────────────────────────────────────────────────────

Consider: A Japanese study published in *Life Sciences* found that a natural substance in raspberries, called ketones, prevented an increase in overall body fat and visceral fat, the deep internal belly fat considered to be the most damaging type of body fat. Ketones are similar to capsaicin, the substance that gives hot peppers their fire. (See page 80 for details about hot peppers.)

Two earlier studies, from the *American Journal of Food Chemistry* and *Food Chemistry*, found that feeding rats berry extracts improved satiety, decreased food intake, and resulted in weight loss and reduced body fat. Berries also are high in fiber, and a German study found that for every gram of fiber we eat, we eliminate 7 calories. In fact, raspberries have one of the best ratios of carbohydrate to fiber. Of the fifteen grams of carbohydrate in one cup of raspberries, eight grams are fiber; that's more than 30 percent of the fiber you need daily.

*Natural Detoxer: Vitamin C.* Vitamin C is a key healing nutrient because it's required for the synthesis of collagen, an important structural part of your blood vessels, tendons, ligaments, and bone. It also plays a role in the production of neurotransmitters, which are critical for healthy brain function and mood regulation. In addition, vitamin C produces carnitine, a molecule essential for fat burning, and it's a powerful antioxidant. Even in small amounts, vitamin C can protect your body's cells from premature aging and disease, and it can regenerate other antioxidants, such as vitamin E. One cup of raspberries provides over 50 percent of your daily vitamin C needs.

*Health Bonus:* Eating berries—about one cup a day—may also protect against early hardening of the arteries, research shows. In a twelve-week European study, hamsters fed raspberry juice had up to a 95 percent reduction in fat deposits in their arteries. That same cup of raspberries may also slow down aging in your brain, according to research under way at Tufts University. That makes sense, since raspberries rank as one of the top ten anti-inflammatory fruits, and inflammation is one of the known causes of dementia.

Berries also reduce the risk of heart disease, cancer, osteoporosis, macular degeneration (the top cause of age-related vision loss), and type 2 diabetes, and boost immune protection.

*Stock Up:* Raspberries are among the most perishable fruits, so it's important to buy fresh berries at their peak. Look for firm, plump berries. If they're at all soft or mushy, they can become moldy within a few hours. Whether you buy them loose at your farmer's market or in a prepackaged container, protect them from getting crushed or wet—both conditions will cause rapid deterioration. Store raspberries in the refrigerator after removing any with signs of mold.

There is nothing more flavorful than a fresh, in-season raspberry, but just as with spinach, fresh isn't your only option. You can use frozen berries as long as they have no added ingredients.

Fact ————————————————————————————————

Are you getting enough magnesium, a mineral involved in more than three hundred bodily reactions? One study found that increasing one's daily intake of magnesium by just 100 mg resulted in a 1 percent increase in bone density. One ounce of almonds packs 80 mg of magnesium; a half cup of cooked spinach, 75 mg.

## seven steps to freezing fresh spinach and raspberries

If you come across some gorgeous greens or berries at your local farmer's market, snatch them up and freeze what you don't use. Freezing is a great way to take advantage of your local bounty in season and save money through the chillier months of the year. Both spinach and raspberries keep for about six months in the freezer.

The trick to preserving the flavor, color, and nutritional value of greens is to follow these seven steps. Skip steps three and four for berries.

1. Wash spinach leaves or berries.
2. Discard any that are moldy or wilted.
3. Immerse in hot water for one minute.
4. Cool.
5. Place on tray or cookie sheet in a single layer, berries or leaves not touching, so they don't fuse together.
6. Freeze on tray for thirty minutes.
7. Transfer into freezer bags.

## incredible eggs

Eggs are a proven weight-loss food. Several studies have compared bagel breakfasts with egg breakfasts and concluded that for weight control, eggs are the better choice.

For example, a University of Connecticut study found that when egg breakfasts and bagel breakfasts contained an identical number of calories, participants who ate the egg breakfasts consumed fewer calories following breakfast, ate fewer total calories in the twenty-four-hour period

## whole eggs won't hurt your heart

For years, health experts counseled people to avoid egg yolks because they're high in cholesterol. (All of the cholesterol in an egg is found in its yolk.) But newer research has confirmed that people on a diet low in saturated fat and adequate in healthful fats can eat one or two whole eggs a day without measurable changes in their blood-cholesterol levels. More than two hundred studies carried out over the past twenty-five years have investigated the relationship between diet and blood-cholesterol levels, and the studies clearly show that saturated fat in the diet, not dietary cholesterol, is what influences blood cholesterol levels the most.

after breakfast, and reported feeling less hungry and more satisfied for up to three hours after the egg-based meal.

A similar study published in the *International Journal of Obesity* found that eating eggs for breakfast as part of a reduced-calorie diet helped overweight dieters lose 65 percent more weight and feel more energized than those who ate a bagel breakfast that had an equal number of calories and an identical volume. But won't eggs raise your levels of "bad" cholesterol? Actually, no. This study found no significant cholesterol differences between the two groups.

Yet another bagel-versus-egg breakfast study found that after eight weeks, egg eaters lost almost twice as much weight, had an 83 percent greater decrease in their waistlines, and reported greater improvements in their energy level. Again, no significant differences were seen in the cholesterol or triglyceride levels in either group, confirming what other studies have shown: healthy people can safely enjoy whole eggs without increasing their risk of heart attack.

*Natural Detoxer: Choline.* Studies have shown that more than 90 percent of Americans are deficient in choline, a nutrient found in eggs that is needed to produce the membrane of each of your body's 100 trillion cells. Eggs are among the best sources; one egg supplies 25 percent of the Daily Value. Choline also is a precursor to acetylcholine, an important neurotransmitter needed for brain health, muscle control, memory, and many other functions. Choline helps your nerves communicate with your muscles; quells inflammation, a known trigger of aging and disease; and prevents the buildup of homocysteine, an amino acid tied to heart disease and stroke risk. According to a Greek study published in the *American Journal of Clinical Nutrition,* people whose diets supplied the highest average intake of choline had inflammatory markers that were at least 20 percent lower than those with the lowest average intakes. Choline also has been shown to block fat absorption and break down fatty deposits in the body.

> I was happy with every single meal I had today!
> KARLA, AGE 34

*Health Bonus:* The protein in eggs ranks highest, among all foods, in biological value; in other words, more protein gets absorbed and incorporated into the body's protein tissues from eggs than from any other food. The biological value of a whole egg is a perfect one hundred, compared to ninety for cow's milk and about seventy-five for fish and chicken.

*Stock Up:* I highly recommend buying USDA-certified organic eggs. Organic eggs come from hens fed an all-vegetarian diet of certified organic grains grown without synthetic pesticides and fertilizers, and the chickens have been given no growth hormones or antibiotics. The eggs can be brown or white. Though brown eggs may appear "healthier," in truth the shell's color is related only to the breed of the chicken, not the quality or nutritional value of the egg. For more information about how organic foods support weight loss, see page 201.

In the recipes I provide, you will see that in the scramble and salad I include the option of eating one whole large organic egg or the whites from three eggs. Based on nutrition research, I believe that eating up to two whole eggs per day is healthful (see the box titled "Whole Eggs Won't Hurt Your Heart" on page 46), but if you dislike egg yolks, or you've been told to follow a low-cholesterol diet by your doctor, stick with egg whites instead. Three whites provide about the same number of calories and protein as one whole egg, without any cholesterol. Another option: buy a carton of organic liquid egg whites instead of cracking the eggs and discarding the yolks yourself.

If you buy eggs by the carton, store them in the refrigerator in their original container. Transferring them to the door of your refrigerator can cause them to absorb odors, lose nutrients, and be exposed to higher temperatures. Also, it's not a good idea to wash eggs before you store them, since this can wash away the protective coating surrounding the shell that keeps bacteria out.

## luscious, lip-smacking yogurt

Yogurt isn't just a healthy snack; it's a weight-loss weapon. In a University of Tennessee study published in the *International Journal of Obesity*, obese men and women were put on a reduced-calorie diet that included three daily portions of yogurt. Compared with dieters assigned the same number of calories but few or no dairy products, the yogurt eaters lost 61 percent more fat and 81 percent more belly fat over a three-month period. They also retained more of their metabolism-revving lean muscle mass.

Fermented dairy foods such as yogurt also are a source of probiotics, the "friendly" bacteria found in yogurt. One of these bacteria is acidophilus, which may be a hidden factor in weight control. Some experts maintain that probiotics help control weight by changing the bacteria in the digestive system. Obese people have been found to carry digestive bacteria that tend to extract more calories from meals, making it easier for them to store excess calories as body fat. When scientists transfer the gastrointestinal (GI) bacteria found in obese mice into their lean counterparts, the skinny mice gain weight, even without additional calories.

That discovery has led researchers to believe that probiotics can produce bacteria that positively impact metabolism and weight control; and one of the best ways to benefit from these "good bugs" is to include yogurt in your diet.

*Natural Detoxer: Probiotics.* Weight control isn't the only potential benefit from probiotics. These bugs are similar to the natural bacteria found in our "guts," and they typically come from two groups: lactobacillus or bifidobacterium. Having enough in your GI tract is vital to your immune system and also aids digestion. Having too few (or too many bad bacteria without enough good to counter them) has been linked to irritable bowel syndrome, infections, and even tooth decay. For years scientists have been studying probiotics' ability to fight allergies and treat diarrhea, urinary- and respiratory-tract illnesses, antibiotic-resistant infections, and eczema. They're also being studied as a form of preventive medicine. A recent Swedish study found that employees given lactobacillus got sick less often and missed far fewer days of work.

Lactobacillus in particular has been shown to lessen the inflammation of arthritis, according to a study published in the *Journal of Nutrition.* In two animal experiments, lab animals fed yogurt with lactobacillus had the least amount of arthritic inflammation, whereas milk had no effect. At this time, there are no standard recommendations about probiotics, including exactly how much to take, how often, for how long, and in what form, but I recommend including probiotic-rich foods in your daily diet. Some studies show that it takes about fourteen days of continuous consumption for the effects to kick in, so eating just one yogurt won't do the trick.

*Health Bonus:* Eating just six ounces of yogurt a day has been shown to slash levels of hydrogen sulfide, which is responsible for bad breath. Yogurt may also wipe out the bacteria that coats your tongue, reducing

> 24 25 26 27 28 29 30
>
> I am so glad I did the full 5-Day Fast Forward. I feel like it just gave me the jump start I needed. I think it also helped me enjoy the Cinch! food that much more and realize how flavorful food can be.
>
> LAURENE, AGE 36

the formation of dental plaque and thereby cutting the risk of cavities and gingivitis.

*Stock Up:* These days you'll find dozens of choices in the yogurt aisle. Some are loaded with sugars, colors, and flavorings; others are pure and natural. Here are my five rules for cutting through the clutter to pick the healthiest container of dairy yogurt. If you don't eat dairy, soy and coconut-milk yogurts (see pages 51 and 52) are great alternatives. They contain less protein but are made the same way, just using soy milk or coconut milk in place of cow's milk.

1. Look for nonfat or 0 percent yogurt, which is made with skim milk. That means all the saturated fat and most of the cholesterol has been skimmed off, but all the protein and calcium remain. Any plain nonfat organic yogurt is fine, but I recommend giving organic 0 percent Greek yogurt and *skyr* (Icelandic) yogurt a try. These yogurts use centuries-old straining processes that remove the whey (liquid), making them thicker and creamier without providing any fat. Plus, they pack up to three times more protein than traditional yogurt. Technically *skyr* is a soft cheese, but its texture and nutrients are similar to Greek yogurt, and it includes the same basic ingredients: skim milk and live active cultures. If you can't find Greek or *skyr* in your local market, stick with plain nonfat organic yogurt. Check the ingredients: you should see only pasteurized nonfat milk and live active cultures such as *L. acidophilus, B. bifidus, S. thermophilus, and L. bulgaricus.*

2. Choose plain over flavored yogurt. It's so much more versatile, and you can sweeten it yourself by adding your own fruit and spices. Plus, many flavored yogurts use artificial sweeteners, which as you now know I oppose, or unnecessary added sugars. Because you'll be combining yogurt with berries during the Fast Forward, you'll be adding all-natural sweetness to balance out the yogurt's tartness.

3. Don't worry that plain yogurt contains sugar. When a cow is

## the skinny on coconut yogurt

Coconut products are flooding the market these days. First there was coconut water, then coconut milk (sold in milk cartons next to the soy milk and organic milk), and now coconut-milk yogurt. This decadent nut used to be considered a major no-no because of its high content of saturated fat, but it now enjoys a serious health halo.

Coconut yogurt contains two important parts of the coconut: the milk, and healthy oils. Several studies have found that coconut oil may aid weight loss because the type of fat it contains, called medium-chain triglycerides (MCTs), is metabolized differently than fats from other oils.

A recent Brazilian study tested the effects of about one ounce of either soybean oil or coconut oil over a twelve-week period with women who were instructed to follow a balanced diet and walk for fifty minutes a day. Body mass index decreased in both groups, but only the coconut-oil eaters experienced a reduction in waist circumference. They also had higher levels of HDL cholesterol, the "good" kind, which helps clear cholesterol deposits from arteries, and had lower ratios of LDL to HDL.

An eight-week study published in the *European Journal of Clinical Nutrition* found that medium-chain fatty acids reduced body weight, body fat, and waist circumference in women with high blood triglycerides. Other research has found that, compared with other oils, coconut oil added to the diets of overweight people helps boost calorie and fat burning and weight loss.

Most of the fat in this delicious oil is saturated, but more and more research confirms that not all saturated fats are villains, and coconut provides antioxidants similar to those in berries, grapes, and dark chocolate. Coconut-milk yogurt is made in the same way as cow's-milk yogurt, using healthful probiotic bacteria. You'll find it in nearly every health-food store and many mainstream markets.

milked, each cup naturally contains about thirteen grams of sugar, called lactose. When milk is made into yogurt, some of that sugar is removed, but even when no sugar has been added in, a six-ounce container will still contain between six and nine grams of sugar.

It's all-natural sugar combined with protein, so it won't wreak havoc with your blood-sugar levels or stoke your appetite.

4. Look for the words *live cultures* and *active cultures* on the label. All yogurts start out with live cultures, but some are heated after the cultures are added, which destroys them, and others may be made with low levels of cultures. The good bacteria in live cultures, also known as probiotic bacteria, have been shown to help keep your digestive system healthy and boost your immune system.

5. Go organic. Organic yogurt is made from hormone-free and antibiotic-free cows fed a pesticide-free diet, and organic dairy products have been shown to contain higher amounts of antioxidants than nonorganic varieties. I believe organic yogurt is worth the extra money.

## slimming soy—an alternative for vegans

If you don't eat eggs or dairy, you can choose organic, soy-based alternatives to eggs and yogurt. In fact, even if you're not vegetarian or vegan, you may enjoy choosing soy yogurt or tofu in place of yogurt and eggs for some of the meals in this plan. Never tried tofu? It's very mild and takes on the flavor of whatever you season it with. Soy yogurt has a slightly nutty flavor, and soy milk, which it's made from, provides about the same amount of protein, calcium, and vitamin D as cow's milk.

In addition to being an excellent source of high-quality, animal-free protein, soy also boasts weight-control benefits. A recent study published in the *European Journal of Nutrition* looked at the relationship of soy intake and body weight throughout the lifetimes of over fourteen hundred Caucasian, Japanese, and Native Hawaiian adults. The scientists found that over a five-year period, higher soy intakes were related to a lower body-mass index. Another study, published in the journal *Endocrinology,* concluded that antioxidants in soy called isoflavones can help you stay lean by reducing the production of fat cells and keeping them

## say no to GMO

GMO stands for *genetically modified organism*. GMOs are products of a relatively new science that allows DNA from one species to be injected into another species to create combinations of plant, animal, bacteria, and viral genes that don't occur in nature or through traditional crossbreeding methods.

In Europe, all food products whose ingredients contain more than 0.9 percent GMOs are labeled as such by the government. In the United States and Canada, consumers aren't informed about which foods contain GMOs, and it's estimated that GMOs may be present in more than 75 percent of the processed foods in your average grocery store.

Polls consistently show that a significant majority of North Americans want to be able to tell whether the food they're purchasing contains GMOs. A 2008 CBS News poll found that 87 percent of consumers want GMOs labeled, and according to a recent CBS/New York Times poll, 53 percent say they wouldn't buy a food if they knew it had been genetically modified.

The biggest concern for most consumers and many food experts is the potential for health risks, including possible allergic reactions and hidden illnesses. A Cornell University study showed that a gene for a bacterial toxin added to corn proved poisonous to monarch butterfly larvae that ate the leaves from those plants. Scientists say it's unclear what unintended effects there may be on foods designed to resist bacteria or pests, or how these foods could upset various balances in nature.

Environmentalists also are concerned that GMOs create the potential for superweeds, superpests, and uncontrolled cross-pollination. University of Chicago researchers were recently awarded a grant to investigate how food allergies are triggered. The study, which was funded by the Environmental Protection Agency, could lay the groundwork for assessing whether GMO crops are more likely to cause food allergies—a question that many consumers have been asking. If you're concerned about GMOs or you'd like to avoid them, look for USDA-certified organic foods, which must not contain genetically modified ingredients.

smaller. In animal studies, those fed soy had decreases in fat production ranging from 37 percent to 57 percent compared with those given standard feed. In humans, a comparable amount of isoflavones could easily be consumed by eating just a few servings of tofu or soy milk per day.

*Health Bonus:* Aside from being cholesterol-free and low in saturated fat, soy is rich in antioxidants and minerals and can be a good source of fiber. Soy foods have also been shown to lower the risk of heart disease, knock down high blood pressure, control blood-sugar and insulin levels, strengthen bones, lower the risk of type 2 diabetes, and slash the risk of certain cancers including those of the breast, endometrium, and prostate.

*Stock Up:* I recommend only USDA-certified organic foods made from whole soybeans. Organic soy cannot be produced by using synthetic pesticides, fertilizers, and herbicides and cannot use genetically modified organisms, or GMOs. (For more on GMOs, see the box "Say No to GMO" on page 53.) There are several nationally available brands of plain organic soy yogurt on the market, so you should easily find it at health-food stores and many mainstream markets.

If you're not familiar with tofu, know that it's simply bean curd. An acidic ingredient (usually *nigari,* the liquid remaining after the salt has been removed from seawater) is added to soy milk, which causes it to coagulate, much like a cooked egg. It's then pressed into blocks. Firm tofu has more of the water pressed out, so it holds its shape better and can be sliced, cubed, or crumbled. That's why firm or extra-firm tofu is a better bet than soft or silken tofu for the meals in this plan.

## the fantastic five

These five foods are amazing superfoods with proven benefits for both health and healthy weight loss. But in the Fast Forward plan, the best

## is soy safe?

Soy has become so popular that these days you can find a soy version of just about any food, from bacon to ice cream. But at the same time, there's been some buzz about a possible link between soy and cancer risk. What's the deal?

The safety of soy depends on whether you're eating whole soy foods, such as organic versions of tofu, soy milk, and plain soy yogurt, or processed soy foods, like fake meats. In a study published in *Carcinogenesis*, scientists gave various soy products to laboratory animals with estrogen-dependent breast tumors. In the animals fed soy flour, comparable to whole soy foods, the tumors did not grow. But the tumors did grow in the animals given pure isoflavones, the antioxidants found in soy. Based on the results, the scientists recommend avoiding processed soy products, like faux meats or bars made with isolated soy components, since these often contain much higher amounts of isoflavones than those found in whole soy foods.

I agree. Taking antioxidants out of a food and consuming them in concentrated doses is something entirely different from eating them in naturally occurring amounts. But I do believe that whole soy foods are safe to eat in moderation, and up to a few servings a day can help you lower your risk of heart disease, type 2 diabetes, high blood pressure, and certain cancers, including breast, endometrial, and prostate cancer.

Whole soy is a good source of high-quality protein, contains no cholesterol, and is low in saturated fat and high in iron and other minerals. Whole soy also contains natural substances that help relax blood vessels, opening up circulation and reducing blood pressure. Just be sure to look for USDA-certified organic soy foods made with whole soy beans.

benefit is that they combine in so many delicious, satisfying ways that they make weight loss easy. Even with the same basic ingredients, the scramble is so different from the salad and the parfait such a different sensory experience compared with the smoothie. Even while you're limiting your food intake, you're exciting your senses and exposing your body to a broad spectrum of powerful nutrients. With just these five foods, you're giving your body a simple prescription for a vigorous nutrient rush, ramping up your health while slimming down your physique.

## what to expect during the *fast forward*

Certainly every person will respond to the 5-Day, 5-Food Fast Forward in a unique fashion, but here, in general, is what you can expect each day, based on comments I have received from numerous people who have rapidly lost weight beginning with the Fast Forward.

24 25 26 27 28 29 30 31 32 33 34 35 36 37

## MY STORY

### Adina Friedman, 28 | Pounds lost in 5 days: 8

## I Lost 1.5 Inches from My Hips in 5 Days!

I had been struggling with my weight, and I was having a really hard time getting motivated. I knew that if I had a more structured plan I'd have a higher chance of succeeding. Before the Fast Forward I always tried to eat healthy, but "trying" and "doing" are two different things. I let a lot of little things (desserts, etc.) slide, and they start adding up. I was eating about three meals a day with snacks throughout the day. Breakfast and lunch were usually pretty healthy, but going out to dinner and getting takeout were unpredictable.

On day one I was surprised by how filling the scramble was. It really seemed like a decent portion size, and I felt fulfilled after the meal. My second meal was the parfait, and while I don't love the taste of plain yogurt, the cinnamon really helped. The salad was the meal I was most worried about. I usually have the least control at dinnertime and end up overeating—but I didn't. And it was

## day 1

On the first day, your body will be trying to figure out what's going on. You'll be fueling yourself with foods, quantities, and combinations that are different from what you are accustomed to. But even though you'll be eating significantly less food than usual, you shouldn't feel overly hungry. That's because you'll be nourishing yourself with foods that keep you fuller longer and better regulate your blood-sugar and insulin levels, and you'll be eating on a set schedule. I'm betting that you'll feel more energetic than you have in weeks.

really nice to not feel stuffed after dinner. Plus I still had the smoothie to look forward to! That evening I found the smoothie to be very refreshing! It was also thick and filling, like a late-night dessert. The almond butter really added a nice flavorful taste and honestly, I probably could have not finished the whole thing.

The next morning the scramble was so easy since I already knew what to do. I added a little bit of minced garlic for flavor, and it was delicious. The raspberries were great with cinnamon too, and the parfait is easy. Day two was Saturday and I was out with my friends, so I packed the salad with me for dinner. My friends wanted to go out and I knew I couldn't go, but I was in a good mood because I felt like I was on my way to looking good and being healthy! Plus the balsamic vinegar was great!

On day three I woke up energized after a good night's sleep. It was Sunday and I was going to miss out on brunch, but I was excited to be doing this. By day five I was still enjoying the food, especially the scramble for breakfast, and at the end of the day the smoothie still really hit the spot.

This experience showed me that I could take charge. In the past it always seemed too hard, but to me the Fast Forward wasn't hard. The hardest thing was just committing to doing it in the first place. I kept my promise to myself that I could succeed. I planned ahead and I didn't cheat or take shortcuts. I can't even believe that I lost eight pounds in just five days!!

By the end of the day, you should feel noticeably "lighter," and by the time you go to sleep you'll feel relief from the sluggishness you may have been experiencing before you started the plan. That's exciting, because it's the beginning of an important dialogue between you and your body!

## day 2

On day two, you'll be much more in touch with the sensation of hunger. I know that hunger can trigger feelings of apprehension. A slight grumbling in your stomach may remind you of previous failed attempts at dieting, when you deprived yourself too much, only to binge later on. But keep the faith: this time is different, because you aren't depriving yourself; you're nourishing your body with healthy foods and allowing yourself to feel the natural, normal sensation of hunger. This is something you might not have felt in a long time, perhaps not even since early childhood.

From the time you were a toddler, you were taught to shut off the physical internal "thermostat" that had been guiding your eating. You began to respond to external cues and imposed food "rules," such as eating because food has been offered or because it's time to eat, or you started to eat for reward, pleasure, or entertainment. Maybe you were given a box of crackers to keep you quiet in the shopping cart while Mom pushed you down the aisles of the supermarket. Maybe you received M&M's as a reward for potty training. In preschool, you probably had a calendar full of birthday parties with cake and ice cream as the main event.

At around this age, you also learned to place foods in certain categories. You've probably seen a two- or three-year-old lunge toward a food she recognizes as comforting or especially yummy, like candy, but turn her nose up at a green bean. That's largely because the adults around her have presented candy as a treat and green beans as a chore—or even a necessary evil. Our culture imbues many unhealthy foods with special powers—a habit that later on undermines healthy eating. From a very young age, you learned to tune out the eating signals your body was sending and unconsciously act on the ones coming from your mind. The 5-Day, 5-Food Fast Forward is an important step toward rewiring those signals.

By day two, you will begin the process of tuning back in to your body's physical sensations of hunger and learning to trust them. This is incredibly powerful, because your body would never direct you to eat in a way that would put your health at risk or keep you overweight.

## day 3

On day three, you'll probably see a noticeable change in your body. Here's why: when you step on a scale, your total weight is a measure of seven distinct entities: muscle, bone, organs (such as your lungs, heart, and liver), fluids (including blood), body fat, the waste inside your digestive tract that you haven't yet eliminated, and glycogen (the form of carbohydrate you sock away in your liver and muscles as a backup fuel). By day three, the water you'll be drinking will help flush out sodium and retained water. (When your water intake has been inconsistent, your body tends to hang on to fluid, but when your body is consistently hydrated, it doesn't feel the need to stock up.) You'll shed excess carbohydrate stores, and the consistency of your meals will stimulate your digestive system to eliminate waste.

By the end of day three, you should feel debloated, and you'll probably notice that your face looks less puffy and your clothes are looser, especially through your hips, belly, and thighs.

## day 4

If the changes I described for day three haven't happened yet, you should feel them by today. At this point, after four days of consistent eating, your body will settle into your new pattern. Because of this, you may feel stronger hunger signals within an hour of your scheduled mealtime. If this happens, don't panic! Mild to moderate hunger is actually normal, and it's something you should experience when you wake up and about three more times during each day, every three to five hours.

Mild to moderate hunger involves distinct physical symptoms, such as a gnawing feeling in your tummy that's usually accompanied by rumbling. There's actually a medical name for the growling noises: borborygmi. The muscles of your stomach and small intestines are constantly contracting, but when your stomach is empty, you can hear gas being shifted around.

Within an hour of your scheduled meal, you may also feel a slight dip in your energy level. That's a sign that your body has used up the fuel you provided at the last meal and is ready for more. This slight energy drain is normal, too.

What isn't normal: severe hunger symptoms, such as difficulty concentrating, dizziness, shakiness, extreme irritability, or mood changes. If you experience these symptoms, your body is short on fuel, and you should double the egg or yogurt portion of each meal to better stabilize your blood sugar.

## day 5

By the last day of the Fast Forward, you should be experiencing a whole new sense of body awareness. In addition to waking up hungry and feeling hungry again within about one hour of each scheduled mealtime, you should feel an even, sustained level of energy between meals. Your digestive system should feel more "regular." That means less irritation and bloating, and a relief from constipation.

By day five, you also should notice that you no longer crave salty, fatty, or sweet foods, and you'll begin to appreciate and savor the natural flavors in your whole-foods diet. By the end of day five, most of my clients are amazed that the thought of eating onion rings or a highly processed energy bar has simply lost its appeal. They can't imagine going back to their morning bear claw or lunchtime burger and fries.

Several of my clients have described themselves as "feeling detoxed without feeling deprived." In just five days, you'll have reset your body!

From this point on, you'll maintain your four-meals-a-day schedule, continue eating at the same times, and enjoy the same beverages, but you'll be ready to move forward with an expanded variety of foods.

## 5-day diary

One of the most important tools in this five-day process is an intimate food diary. Think of your diary as a conversation with yourself, or even a conversation between you and me. You'll notice that I ask you to record in your 5-Day Diary not only what and how much you ate and drank, but also insights about how you feel physically and emotionally. Physically,

### sip your stress away

A Japanese study published in the *American Journal of Clinical Nutrition*, conducted with over forty thousand people, found that levels of psychological stress were 20 percent lower in those who drank at least five cups of green tea per day compared with those who drank less than one cup per day. The results held true even after accounting for factors such as age, sex, medical history, body mass index, alcohol consumption, cigarette smoking, and diet. A previous Japanese study reported that green tea extracts were effective in offsetting the physical and mental fatigue associated with stress.

Fact ───────────────────────────────────────────────
Women in the highest 25 percent of optimism scores had a 9 percent lower risk of
developing heart disease and a 14 percent lower chance of dying, period, over an eight-
year span. Those with the most cynical scores were 16 percent more likely to die from
any cause.
─────────────────────────────────────────────────────

tune in to how your body is responding. For example, one of my clients
told me the Fast Forward meals made her feel "light on her feet." Another said that during the Fast Forward her digestive system felt "less
swollen and irritated."

The 5-Day Diary consists of pages of three columns each. The first
column asks about your meals and meal times. The second column, titled
"Physical Signs," is there to help you learn how your muscles, digestive
system, hormones, and so on—the physical you—respond to a simple,
fresh, clean eating plan. The third column, "Emotional Signs," asks you
to explore your emotional reactions. How does it feel to free yourself
from the way you were eating before you started this plan? What are you
learning about your relationship with food?

At the bottom of each daily diary page, I included what I call an
"Insighter Question." I know that these questions aren't easy, and your
first reaction may be "I don't know." But take some time to think them
through. The answers will come to you, and by writing them down you'll
begin to untangle your old patterns and build healthy, new ones that will
last.

I've included all this because making lasting change requires more
than just following an eating plan. Life's not that simple. There are dozens
of things that we all know we "should" be doing every day but don't—get
eight hours of sleep, floss our teeth, slather on sunscreen, and so on. Not
knowing what to do isn't what holds most people back. The greatest bar-
rier is not being able or ready to change.

I've met so many really smart, amazing, dynamic people—probably
just like you—who just get stuck. That's part of being human, and my
number one message to someone who finds herself there is to get really,

really honest about what's going on and why, and vow not to beat your-self up about it. It's never too late to make changes. Even if you've been stuck in a rut for years, you can break free and look and feel better within days. In workshops, I've asked women to say exactly what they're think-ing while looking in a mirror. They typically don't want to, partly because it's so private, partly because saying it seems more harsh than thinking it. But facing the thoughts in your head is important, because even when unspoken, they deeply affect how you feel. Negative self-talk leads to negative emotions, which can trigger depression or cause you to want to punish yourself or cope in an unhealthy way, like starving yourself, binge eating, or allowing others to mistreat you.

Throughout this process, if you catch yourself being negative in your mind, stop and ask yourself, "Would I say that out loud to my best friend?" Focus on treating yourself the way you would treat the person you love and care about the most. I know it's not something you can transform overnight, but switching your self-talk is one of the keys to changing your relationship with food and your health.

As you fill out your diary, commit to a policy of no negative self-talk. These questions are not meant to shame you or make you feel bad or guilty—just the opposite. The goal is for you to learn, openly and hon-estly, about yourself, without judgment, so you can get "unstuck" and move forward in a way that's healthy, both mentally and physically.

This five-day process will allow you to gain an incredible level of awareness, which will foster a sense of change from within—not because you "should," and not even because you want to, but because it feels right.

## the 5-day diary

# day 1

| Meal: *Fill in food, beverages, quantity, and time consumed.* | Physical signs: *What is your body telling you? Do you feel full, satisfied, energized? How is your body responding to its fresh start?* | Emotional signs: *What is your mind telling you? What are you learning about your relationship with food?* |
|---|---|---|
| Scramble Time: | | |
| Parfait Time: | | |
| Salad Time: | | |
| Smoothie Time: | | |

INSIGHTER QUESTION: A recent study found that 70 percent of adults would not want their children to adopt their eating habits because they don't believe they set a good example. Do you fall into that group? Tonight, make two lists: (1) "Personal unhealthy eating patterns I'd like to change and why" and (2) "Habits I feel represent a healthy relationship with food."

_____

_____

_____

_____

# day 2

| Meal: *Fill in food, beverages, quantity, and time consumed.* | Physical signs: *What is your body telling you? Do you feel full, satisfied, energized? How is your body responding to its fresh start?* | Emotional signs: *What is your mind telling you? What are you learning about your relationship with food?* |
|---|---|---|
| Scramble Time: | | |
| Parfait Time: | | |
| Salad Time: | | |
| Smoothie Time: | | |

INSIGHTER QUESTION: Studies show that 75 percent of Americans don't eat the minimum recommended number of servings of fruits and vegetables, and 90 percent don't meet the minimum for whole grains. What gets in your way? List all the "real life" obstacles that interfere with your ability to consistently eat healthfully.

_____

_____

_____

_____

_____

# day 3

| Meal: *Fill in food, beverages, quantity, and time consumed.* | Physical signs: *What is your body telling you? Do you feel full, satisfied, energized? How is your body responding to its fresh start?* | Emotional signs: *What is your mind telling you? What are you learning about your relationship with food?* |
|---|---|---|
| Scramble Time: | | |
| Parfait Time: | | |
| Salad Time: | | |
| Smoothie Time: | | |

INSIGHTER QUESTION: Do you find yourself reaching for food when you're bored, tired, overwhelmed, or sad? How does using food to feed your emotions make you feel physically and mentally? Are you aware that you're eating emotionally in the moment? What activities help you escape, detach, or vent that don't involve eating?

_____

_____

_____

_____

_____

# day 4

| Meal: *Fill in food, beverages, quantity, and time consumed.* | Physical signs: *What is your body telling you? Do you feel full, satisfied, energized? How is your body responding to its fresh start?* | Emotional signs: *What is your mind telling you? What are you learning about your relationship with food?* |
| --- | --- | --- |
| Scramble Time: | | |
| Parfait Time: | | |
| Salad Time: | | |
| Smoothie Time: | | |

INSIGHTER QUESTION: On a scale from zero to ten (ten being highest), rank how important having good health is to you. Do you feel that your daily habits correspond to your ranking? For example, a lot of my clients rank their health as a nine or ten, but on a day-to-day basis, healthy eating becomes a low priority for them. Does this tend to be the case for you? If so, why?

_____

_____

_____

_____

# day 5

| Meal: *Fill in food, beverages, quantity, and time consumed.* | Physical signs: *What is your body telling you? Do you feel full, satisfied, energized? How is your body responding to its fresh start?* | Emotional signs: *What is your mind telling you? What are you learning about your relationship with food?* |
|---|---|---|
| Scramble Time: | | |
| Parfait Time: | | |
| Salad Time: | | |
| Smoothie Time: | | |

INSIGHTER QUESTION: Do you see eating healthfully as something you "should" do or something you want to do? A lot of my clients tell me that they want to eat healthfully, yet something in them rebels, almost like the feeling you had when you were a child and your parents told you that you had to do your homework. How can you reframe healthy eating from a "should" to a "want"? What will eating healthfully give you that's important to you today?

_____

_____

_____

_____

# diary wrap-up

On this final day of your diary, it's important to reflect back on how you were eating one week ago. I know it's been only five days, but what has the Cinch! Fast Forward plan allowed you to learn about yourself, your body, and your emotional connections to food?

The questions included in this diary are meant to open the door to a better understanding of your emotional connections to food, but this is just the beginning. As you continue on for the next twenty-five days, I encourage you to use the tools found in chapter 8. There you'll find a number of exercises designed to dig deeper into your eating triggers that are not related to physical hunger. This chapter can help you systematically identify and replace food with healthier alternatives when it's your mind, rather than your body, that needs to be nourished.

If emotional eating turns out to be one of the greatest hurdles in your ability to successfully change your relationship with food, I believe the information and resources in chapter 8 will help you begin to break the cycle.

# 3

24 25 26 27 28 29 30 31 32 33

# a little SASS
# goes a long way

**B**efore you get started, either on the Fast Forward or Cinch! core plan, I want to introduce you to one of the most unique features of Cinch!, and the one I'm most excited about: *SASS*. This acronym stands for "Slimming And Satiating Seasonings." There are five categories:

- Vinegar
- Citrus juice and zest
- Hot peppers
- Tea
- Herbs and spices

These are the only types of seasonings you will use to flavor your food over the thirty days. At least one of these seasoning categories is included in each meal on the plan. Using these seasonings in every meal is a triple bonus. First, they replace the salt and sugar in recipes without affecting the flavor, so you feel more satisfied eating healthier meals. Second, they contain natural properties that speed weight loss. For an added bonus, they boost your body's defenses against aging and disease.

For these reasons, I believe that the SASS seasonings are the only five types you need—period. They're so rich in flavor, versatile, and energizing that you will hardly miss drowning your salad in ranch dressing or slathering your sandwiches with mayo. Instead of using high-sodium soy sauce in your stir-fry, you'll enjoy the tangy deliciousness of fresh citrus juice blended with vinegar, ginger, and scallions; rather than bathing broccoli or asparagus in butter, you'll toss these veggies in extra-virgin olive oil and a mixture of Italian herbs. On my plan, you'll still get your creamy guacamole—absolutely!—but you will enhance the rich avocado flavor with fresh cilantro, cracked black pepper, diced jalapeños, and wedges of fresh lime.

During the Fast Forward plan, you'll add freshly grated ginger to your smoothie and toss your spinach salad with balsamic vinegar and fresh-squeezed tangerine juice. During the core Cinch! plan, you'll take these seasonings to a new level, folding tangerine zest and basil into your Tangerine Almond Twist, adding a pinch of cloves to your Banana Hazelnut Ricotta Toast, and blending green-tea leaves into your Cherry Almond Smoothie.

For multiple reasons, SASS is the cornerstone of Cinch! If you're feeling creative and want to learn how to build your own meals and experiment with the seasonings yourself, I'll show you how in chapter 6.

## why SASS?

When I left *Prevention* magazine to go back into private practice, I started to cook more often for myself and create quick, healthy recipes for my clients. Around this time, I also began to immerse myself in the groundbreaking research that was being done on the health and weight-

## SASS excess sodium out of your diet

Sodium has been snuck into practically every food product on the market. We're so used to sodium that we don't even realize how much salt drowns out the natural, delicious flavors of fresh food. When you rid your diet of excess sodium, your taste buds come alive, and you experience an avalanche of new flavor sensations, including the subtle, genuine taste of whole foods like fresh corn and of intense seasonings like peppercorn and oregano. Sodium also leads to water retention, so slashing your intake means you'll no longer struggle with puffiness and bloat.

Seasonings help you cut back on the sodium in meals without missing the flavor—a swap that may also add years to your life. A review of seventeen published studies found that even a modest reduction in sodium intake can have a significant effect on blood pressure in people with both high and normal blood pressure. In just four weeks, cutting sodium by 2,400 mg per day slashed the risk of dying from stroke 14 percent among people with high blood pressure and by 9 percent among people with normal blood pressure. The risk of dying from heart disease also was reduced—by 6 percent in the group with hypertension and by 4 percent in the group with normal blood pressure.

Sodium has become the "it" nutritional villain, and reducing our intake to the recommended level could result in 11 million fewer cases of high blood pressure each year.

But sodium is an essential nutrient. We need a certain amount to help nerves and muscles work properly in regulating the balance of fluid in the body. The maximum daily sodium recommendation is 1,500 to 2,300 mg, the typical amount in one can of soup. Yet the average person consumes 3,400 mg per day. About 70 percent of that comes from processed foods such as soups and frozen entrées. That's why the best way to slash your intake is to build your meals from whole, unprocessed foods like the ones I use in this plan, adding flavor by using the SASS salt-free seasonings.

control benefits of some of my favorite seasonings and flavors. I found myself coming back to the same handful of seasonings. I'd sprinkle vinegar on my salad of fresh field greens, tomatoes, and basil. I'd mix citrus juice into my stir-fry sauce, citrus zest into my dark-chocolate truffles. I'd include hot peppers in black beans and use tea to sauté my veggies. I liberally used herbs and spices in everything from my morning coffee to an afternoon fruit smoothie.

This group of seasonings soon became the signature of my meals, and I believe they're the world's best-kept diet secret. There are three scientific reasons that these five seasonings are powerful weight-loss weapons:

1. They are incredibly low in calories but bursting with flavor and aroma. Research shows that adding even small amounts of intense, pleasing flavors to your food can help you feel satisfied on fewer calories and shed dramatic amounts of weight. (More on that later!)
2. They are rich in antioxidants, and fascinating research has linked higher antioxidant intakes with lower body-fat levels, even when calorie intakes are the same.
3. Each has separately been shown in published studies to boost fat burning.

When I bring my lunch to work I pack the vinegar and herbs separately. They travel well!
AMY, AGE 28

## slash calories without sacrificing flavor

A tablespoon of aged balsamic vinegar has a mere 15 calories, one ounce of lime juice 8 calories, a cup of brewed tea just 2 calories, a whole jalapeño 4 calories; and herbs and spices such as mint and turmeric contain zero calories. In contrast, one tablespoon of butter, one tablespoon of mayo, two tablespoons of ketchup, and one-quarter cup of Ranch dressing—condiment amounts that you could easily include in a single day if not a single meal—add up to a whopping 500 calories. A surplus 500 calories a day is enough to pack fifty extra pounds on your frame over one year. Using the five SASS seasonings in place of sauces, condiments, and dressings immediately cuts several hundred calories from your meals while helping trigger your body's "I'm full" mechanism.

Scientists from the Smell and Taste Treatment and Research Foundation in Chicago put this notion to the test by creating various crystals calls "tastants" to enhance a meal's flavor. In a controlled study, over fourteen hundred overweight or obese volunteers were asked to sprinkle the tastants on their food for six months, keeping their diet and exercise routines otherwise unchanged. After six months, those who used the additives lost an average of 30.5 pounds, compared with just 2 pounds for the control group, which used no flavorings. The scientists say that powerful tastes and smells send messages to the brain that cause people to feel fuller faster.

## more antioxidants mean greater weight-loss results

Plant-based foods, including this group of seasonings, are a rich source of antioxidants. Mountains of research have proven that antioxidants play a vital role in antiaging and disease prevention. But only recently has science begun to show that they also help regulate body weight.

University of Florida researchers have developed an index that ranks the number of calories consumed from plant-based foods compared with overall daily calorie intake. It's called the phytochemical index, or PI, score. The term *phytochemical* is often used interchangeably with *antioxidant;* it simply refers to chemical compounds that naturally occur in plants. A totally plant-based, vegan diet (excluding hard liquor and refined sugars) could have a perfect score of 100, whereas a typical American diet, heavy with meat, sugar, and fried foods and low in fruits and veggies, would score below 20. In a study published in the *Journal of Human Nutrition and Dietetics,* the Florida researchers found that people of normal weight had PI scores 10.3 points higher, on average, than overweight or obese people. And even though both groups consumed about the same number of daily calories, those with lower PI scores had higher body mass indexes, larger waist circumferences, and higher body-fat percentages.

In another study, researchers at the Yale School of Medicine found that free radicals—a by-product of normal metabolism whose levels spike when we're under stress—stimulate the brain's appetite center, whereas antioxidants from plant-based foods combat free radicals and thus trigger satiety.

## nature's fat burners

Here's a little more about why each of the five signature seasonings in this plan is essential in helping you lose weight.

### vinegar

When you think of flavoring your food with vinegar, salad may be all that comes to mind. But this lip-puckering condiment can be used in a wide variety of wonderful ways. In this plan, I drizzle balsamic vinegar over strawberry avocado tacos, use it as a marinade for chilled lentil and wild rice salad, and even fold it into chocolate truffles. Vinegar is made by fermenting a number of foods, from grapes (in balsamic vinegar) to rice and apples. For a culinary adventure, you can also use fruit-infused vinegars such as raspberry, fig, and pomegranate.

Considering how much I enjoy the flavor of vinegar, I'm thrilled to tell you about its weight-loss properties. A study from Arizona State University at Tempe, for example, found that people who consumed just a tablespoon of vinegar before lunch and dinner lost an average of two pounds over a four-week period without making any other dietary changes. Another Arizona State study, a research review published in the *Journal of the American College of Nutrition,* found that adding vinegar to meals can help naturally curb calorie intake for the remainder of the day by up to 16 percent, or 200 to 275 calories. This one change alone is enough to trigger a loss of twenty to twenty-eight pounds in a year's time. This is one of the reasons you won't count calories on this plan. As the studies show, the addition of certain ingredients triggers a natural reduction in your food intake.

Acetic acid, the main component of vinegar, seems to have potent health benefits. A Japanese study found that acetic acid helps control blood pressure and blood-sugar levels while curbing fat accumulation. Mice that were fed acetic acid alongside a typical Western-style diet developed less body fat and liver fat than mice that drank water. Liver fat is considered to be an even better marker for diseases like type 2 diabetes and heart disease than belly fat. Significant increases also were seen in the expressions of genes that regulate fat- and calorie-burning proteins.

When the same researchers tested the effects in obese Japanese subjects in a double-blind trial, they found similar results. The volunteers—all with similar BMIs (body mass indexes) and waist circumferences—were randomly assigned to three groups: one group with a daily sixteen-ounce beverage containing one tablespoon of vinegar, a second group with a sixteen-ounce beverage that had two tablespoons of vinegar, and a third group with a sixteen-ounce beverage that had no vinegar. After twelve weeks, the two groups that had vinegar had lower body weights, BMIs, visceral fat (deep internal belly fat), waist measurements, and blood triglyceride levels than the no-vinegar group.

> My body just appreciates this new routine. I have soooo much more energy throughout the day, and I'm not as stressed. I just feel different overall.
>
> LAURENE, AGE 36

There's more: In a small study published in the *European Journal of Clinical Nutrition,* Swedish researchers tested the ability of acetic acid to lower the effects of a bread-based meal on blood-sugar and insulin levels and on satiety. Three types of vinegar with varying levels of acetic acid were served with a portion of white bread containing fifty grams of carbohydrates at breakfast in a random order after overnight fasts. Bread served without vinegar was used as a reference meal. The scientists found that bread with vinegar reduced postmeal levels of blood sugar and insulin and increased the self-reported rates of satiety. The highest acetic level of vinegar significantly lowered blood sugar levels 30 and 45 minutes after the meal and increased satiety for up to 120 minutes.

### citrus juice and zest

Before I moved to New York City, I lived in Florida, where I had a grapefruit tree and an orange tree in my backyard that produced so much fruit I gave away dozens of bags each season. With so much citrus to experiment with, I learned a few important lessons. First, a little juice goes a long way. Juice is concentrated, so an eight-ounce glass of OJ is the equivalent of about four fresh oranges—far more than you'd eat in one sitting—and a high dose of calories.

An ounce of orange juice, however, can add to a vinaigrette dressing just enough sweetness, an intense layer of flavor, and a perfect measure of fragrant aroma. Also, zest is like the icing on the citrus cake! For many years I discarded citrus rind like a banana peel, not appreciating the fact that it was laden with such delicious, nutrient-rich seasoning. Zesting is easy to do, and a sprinkling of freshly grated or dried citrus rind can be used in everything from water and tea to yogurt and spaghetti squash. You'll find recipes using the combinations I just mentioned and more in chapter 4, such as the Zesty Cranberry Walnut Parfait at breakfast, Strawberry Walnut "Ice Cream" with Lime Zest snack, and Edamame Cashew Ginger Stir-Fry, which includes a sauce made from 100 percent orange juice combined with rice vinegar, scallions, and fresh ginger.

Citrus juice is also one of the best sources of vitamin C. A single ounce supplies 120 percent of the Daily Value, and vitamin C is linked to less body fat and smaller waist measurements. Arizona State University researchers found that the amount of vitamin C in the bloodstream is directly related to fat oxidation—the body's ability to use fat as a fuel source—both during exercise and at rest. At the beginning of a trial involving obese men and women, participants with the lowest concentrations of vitamin C in their blood had the highest body-fat mass, and they tended not to burn fat well compared with their less obese counterparts. Fat burning was measured in people with marginal or adequate vitamin C status during a sixty-minute treadmill test. The researchers found that those with poor vitamin C status burned 25 percent less fat during the treadmill test than those with adequate vitamin C status, and fat burning during exercise was enhanced fourfold in people with normal levels. Throughout the study, as some of the participants' blood vitamin C concentrations fell, so did their ability to burn fat—by a whopping 11 percent.

> YUMMY! I love, love, love the almond butter with toast. I think I will eat this every day with some blueberries and milk. Really satisfying too. Easy to prepare.
>
> RENEE, AGE 45

Remarkably, vitamin C isn't the only component in citrus that helps you shed pounds. Naringenin, an antioxidant in the flavonoid family, has been shown to prevent weight gain and other signs of metabolic syndrome, which can lead to type 2 diabetes and increased risk of heart disease, according to research from the University of Western Ontario. Scientists fed one group of mice a high-fat, typically Western diet to bring on the symptoms of metabolic syndrome. A second group was fed the exact same diet supplemented with naringenin, found in oranges and grapefruits. Unlike the mice that weren't supplemented, these mice didn't develop insulin resistance or become obese, their blood-sugar levels completely normalized, and they experienced protective changes in triglyceride and cholesterol levels. The scientists found that naringenin worked by reprogramming the animals' livers to burn excess fat rather than store it. The health of your liver is vital to your body's overall metabolism, including how well you regulate blood-sugar and insulin levels, which are tied to overall fat storage, as well as normal thyroid function. The bottom line is that a hampered liver can affect your body's overall ability to burn fat and calories.

Naringenin is just one of the flavonoids found in citrus. Others include hesperidin, quercitrin, rutin, and tangeritin. No, you don't need to remember these names, but you'll probably remember the phenomenal results of this Dutch study of more than four thousand women aged fifty-five to sixty-nine: over a fourteen-year period, those who consumed more of these antioxidants gained two times less weight than those with the lowest flavonoid intakes.

There's just something about citrus. The vitamin C and antioxidants are probably what set it apart from other fruits as a fat burner, and the results stand up against apple juice. In a twelve-week study published in the *Journal of Medicinal Food*, obese volunteers were divided into four groups: (1) those given placebo capsules and seven ounces of apple juice; (2) those given grapefruit capsules and seven ounces of apple juice; (3) those given eight ounces of grapefruit juice and a placebo capsule; (4) those given half of a fresh grapefruit and a placebo capsule. After twelve weeks, the fresh-grapefruit group lost 3.5 pounds, the grapefruit-juice group lost 3.3 pounds, the grapefruit-capsule group lost 2.4 pounds, and the nongrapefruit group shed less than a pound. Grapefruit eaters also had a significant reduction in blood-sugar and insulin levels after their meals.

The vitamin C and natural antioxidants aren't just in citrus juice; they're also in the rind. A University of Arizona study concluded that eating as little as one tablespoon of citrus zest per week can reduce the risk of squamous-cell carcinoma skin cancer by 30 percent.

When you zest citrus yourself, use organically grown citrus, since conventionally grown fruit has pesticide residues on the skin. Wash and dry the fruit, and use a zester, vegetable peeler, box grater, or microplane to remove the colored part of the peel. Avoid including the white pith beneath the peel, which tastes very bitter. You can chop or dice larger pieces if needed. Larger pieces will stay fresher longer. You can dry fresh zest and store it in a small airtight container for about a month, or wrap and freeze it. Frozen zest will keep about six months.

## hot peppers

My affair with hot peppers began when I met my husband, Jack. He's a Texan who practically breathes fire. I've witnessed him eating not just one but several habanero peppers, the hottest common variety, in a single meal. One of our first meals together was fajitas, and because I was so head-over-heels, I tried to impress him by taking a big bite of his fresh jalapeño—my first.

What happened next wasn't so sexy. My eyes watered, my nose ran, and my lips and tongue were so numb I could barely talk or eat. And as I learned, dousing the flames with water only spreads heat throughout your mouth. Fortunately, Jack found the incident amusing, and throughout our thirteen years together my tolerance for hot peppers has grown— although not quite to Jack's level. I'm now a fan of adding minced jalapeños to my quick-fix guacamole and adding crushed red pepper to beans and barley. In chapter 4 you'll find many meals seasoned with black peppercorn, such as Peppery Kiwi Almond Crunch and the Smoked Gouda and Grilled Onion Salad, but you can also feel free to add a whole or sliced pepper to any meal or enjoy them on the side. Jack often nibbles on a fresh jalapeño, serrano, or chili pepper between bites. In chapter 6, you'll find a list of hot peppers in the SASS section. Try experimenting with milder varieties first, like banana and poblano peppers, and slowly build your tolerance to more potent varieties like cayenne.

But the top reason hot peppers are on my SASS list is because capsaicin, the natural substance that gives them their fire, has been shown to rev up metabolism and whittle waistlines. Studies show that eating about one tablespoon of chopped red or green chili pepper, equal to 30 mg of capsaicin, can temporarily boost metabolism by up to 23 percent.

At the University of Maryland School of Medicine, eighty middle-aged overweight men and women participated in a twelve-week double-blind study to test the effects of capsaicin. The participants were randomly assigned to a capsaicin or placebo group. The researchers found that those in the hot seats lost more weight and abdominal fat than the

## how i SASS up my morning cup of joe

Here's my secret for delicious java: I toss a "teabag" of mulling spices into my coffeemaker every morning. I've loved coffee since I was a kid, but I always had to add sugar to cut the bitterness. I gradually conquered my sugar fix and eventually began enjoying the flavor of good-quality coffee without sweetener, but to give it a kick, I've always sprinkled in cinnamon and nutmeg.

Then one day at the market I spotted a product I hadn't seen before: R. W. Knudsen's Organic Mulling Spices. One box contains twenty-five tea bags filled with cinnamon, cloves, ginger, lemon peel, and orange peel. The next morning when I was making coffee, I saw them in my cupboard and tossed one in with my coffee grounds. My husband said it made our kitchen smell like fall, and it infused a delicious layer of flavor in my brew, not to mention the antioxidants found in these seasonings. Give it a try!

Go to www.rwknudsenfamily.com and type in your zip code to find out where to find this brand at your local market. If it's not available locally, you can purchase it online at amazon.com. You can also sprinkle some spices directly into your coffee grounds. Cinnamon, nutmeg, cloves, and citrus zest all add amazing flavor, and you can also buy blends such as apple-pie spice or pumpkin-pie spice.

placebo group. Among the capsaicin subjects, the scientists also found an increase in fat-burning capacity by the end of the study.

A University of Denmark study published in the *Journal of Biological Chemistry* found that capsaicin can directly induce thermogenesis, the process by which cells convert energy into heat, and thus crank up calorie burning. And Taiwanese researchers found that capsaicin prevented fat cells grown in a laboratory from filling with fat. Another Taiwanese study from the *Journal of Agricultural and Food Chemistry* found evidence that capsaicin can reduce the growth of fat cells. The researchers

I'm wearing a dress that used to be a little snug. Now it fits perfectly!

AMY, AGE 28

tested capsaicin's effects on emerging fat cells grown in laboratory cultures, finding that capsaicin prevented the cells from filling with fat and becoming full-fledged fat cells.

And according to a study from the University of Ulsan in South Korea, dietary intakes of capsaicin, the compound that gives red pepper its heat, may prevent the development of diabeteslike symptoms in obese people. Animals fed a high-fat diet supplemented with just a dash of capsaicin—0.015 percent—lowered blood-sugar insulin levels, according to the findings published in *Obesity*. Scientists say the data suggest that dietary capsaicin may reduce obesity-induced glucose intolerance by not only suppressing inflammatory responses but also enhancing fat burning.

Fact ————————————————————————————————————
The cells of regular tea drinkers have a younger biological age than those of nondrinkers!
————————————————————————————————————————

*tea*

We are not a nation of tea drinkers. Among twenty-five tea-drinking countries, the United States ranks just twentieth in per capita tea consumption. Our average intake is ten to twelve times lower than that of the top three: Turkey, the United Kingdom, and Ireland. But I'm doing all I can to change that!

Tea not only is a fantastic beverage but also can be thought of as a seasoning. Brewed, chilled green tea can be used to sauté, steam, or marinate vegetables, tofu, poultry, or seafood, and tea leaves can be ground in a peppermill with or without other spices as a delicious, aromatic seasoning for everything from stir-fries to fruit and chocolate. In the pages to come you'll find meals such as Green-Tea Chicken with Avocado Corn Salad, a Cherry Almond Green Tea Smoothie, and my signature Green Tea Truffles.

Green, black, white, and oolong tea all come from the same plant.

Black tea is fermented, green and white are not, and oolong is semifermented. Each variety is a rich source of antioxidants that play a role in reducing the risk of various diseases, including Alzheimer's, certain cancers, and heart disease. In addition, tea, the world's most popular beverage, also can help you lose weight!

A Japanese study asked healthy women to drink either water, oolong tea, or green tea, and measured their levels of calorie burning. Compared with the water drinkers, those who drank oolong tea burned 10 percent more calories for up to two hours, and the green-tea drinkers burned 4 percent more calories. A study of men, published in the *Journal of Nutrition*, compared the calorie-burning effects of five daily servings of four beverages over a three-day period: water, full-strength tea, half-strength tea, and water containing 270 mg of caffeine (in order to make sure that there weren't other contributing factors in tea). Calorie burning (which includes burning carbohydrate) increased by 2.9 percent and 3.4 percent for the full-strength tea and caffeinated water, respectively; fat burning spiked by 12 percent in the full-strength tea group.

*Tea: A Major Immune Booster.* I like to refer to tea as medicine in a mug (at least I drink it by the mugful instead of in a dainty teacup). Tea has been shown to boost bone density and slow bone loss, slash the risk of heart disease and cancer, fend off aging, and also give the immune system a boost.

In a study published in the *Proceedings of the National Academy of Sciences,* Harvard scientists found that tea primes your body's immune system against substances called alkylamines, which are commonly present in tea (but not coffee) as well as in some bacteria, parasites, and fungi. Researchers recruited twenty-one non-tea-drinking volunteers and asked them to drink either five to six small cups of black tea or five to six small cups of instant black coffee every day for four weeks. Blood samples taken after tea drinking showed that the volunteers' bodies produced five times more of a crucial antibacterial substance than before they began drinking tea, and coffee drinking had no immune-boosting effect. The scientists concluded that the effect was akin to keeping the body's immune system in a state of readiness so it can react if bacteria or other unwanted invaders do arrive.

## herbs and spices

Fresh mint, basil, oregano, cracked black pepper, freshly grated ginger, cinnamon, cloves, vanilla bean—there are dozens of delectable herbs and spices, each with unique antioxidants, aromas, and flavors. A few have made headlines recently for their weight-control ties.

In a study published in the *American Journal of Clinical Nutrition,* cinnamon was found to slow the rate of stomach emptying after meals and reduce the postmeal rise in blood sugar. I've added cinnamon to many of the meals in this plan, including Apple Pecan Breakfast Pilaf and the Cherry Almond Green Tea Smoothie.

Black pepper, which comes from the berries of the pepper plant, was found to increase calorie burning by stimulating the nervous system as well as the mitochondria—the powerhouses in cells that act like minifurnaces to generate fuel. I fold pepper into my Pineapple Almond Peppercorn Parfait and use it to dust the Mediterranean Lentils over Couscous.

Ginger has also been found to rev up calorie burning, according to the results of animal studies. You'll find it in every stir-fry meal in this plan as well as in the Salmon Ginger Rice Bowl and the Chocolate Pear Ginger Smoothie.

These seasonings can also help you stall the aging process. In a University of Georgia study published in the *Journal of Medicinal Food,* extracts of twenty-four herbs and spices from a local supermarket were tested for their ability to prevent tissue damage and inflammation caused by high levels of blood sugar. In the study, the seasonings inhibited protein glycation, a process in which sugar bonds with proteins to form substances known as advanced glycation end products, or AGE compounds, which are known to contribute to diabetes and aging.

Garlic is my must-have seasoning for Fresh Mozzarella Basil "Pizzalad" and Herbed Walnut Artichoke Lettuce Wraps. Two recent studies,

## SASS superheroes

You've probably heard that blueberries are "superfoods"—foods with extra-powerful doses of natural, disease-fighting compounds. But the truth is, practically every plant-based food on earth is a nutrition superhero, not just the exotic ones, and some of the most potent are seasonings.

Garlic fights viruses, prevents arteries from hardening, and has been linked to a reduced risk of at least seven types of cancer. Herbs and spices are some of the most potent protectors of your health. Studies show that they tend to be higher in antioxidants than fruits and vegetables. You'll find as many antioxidants in one teaspoon of cinnamon as in a half cup of blueberries. This amazing spice has consistently been shown to help control blood-sugar levels and prevent blood clots. Research shows that turmeric, the gorgeous spice found in curry seasoning, fights cancer and Alzheimer's, curbs fat accumulation, and improves the health of your liver and digestive system. Rosemary increases blood flow to the head, improving concentration, keeping the brain younger, and protecting the brain from stroke.

both from the Federation of American Societies for Experimental Biology (FASEB) journal, point to garlic's fat-burning effects. In one Korean study, mice were fed a high-fat diet for eight weeks to induce obesity. They were then put on a maintenance diet supplemented with either 2 percent or 5 percent garlic for another eight weeks. The researchers found that both garlic diets reduced body weights and blood triglycerides. In a second Korean study, mice were again fattened up and then fed a 2 percent or 5 percent garlic-supplemented diet for eight weeks. The body weights of the garlic-fed mice were reduced by 8 percent and 20 percent, respectively, compared with the control diet, and their triglyceride and cholesterol levels dropped as well.

# MY STORY

## Heidi Matzelle, 31  |  Pounds lost: 10

## I Lost Those Last 10 Pounds— Right Before My Wedding!

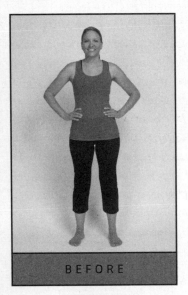

BEFORE

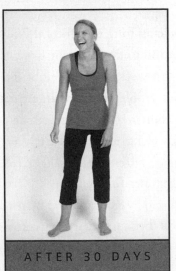

AFTER 30 DAYS

I always tried to eat healthy, but I'd fall into the junk-food trap of eating chips when I was bored or getting offtrack on the weekends. An even bigger issue was portion control. But this year I had the greatest motivation in my life to lose those last ten pounds—tying the knot with the man of my dreams! So when I saw the opportunity to try a weight-loss approach, I submitted my story and photo. And now I'll be walking down the aisle at my goal weight!

Immediately I began to feel energized on this plan, despite drinking only one cup of coffee a day. Cinch! really made me think about what I was putting into my body and how my diet affected my overall health. We get so fixated on the number on the scale as opposed to how we feel and how our bodies are changing in other ways. This plan allowed me to start sleeping a solid seven and a half hours and waking up with some pep in my step. I just feel so good about myself!

The whole month was a learning experience. I learned portion control, and I think that my body is now trained to eat four times a day. I don't have cravings for junk food and don't miss it either. Alcohol is another thing I don't miss. My fiancé, Chris, and I are big boaters. We'd hang out on the boat and enjoy a few beers and I used to have beer or wine when we'd go out on the weekends. Now I'm content drinking my flavored all-natural seltzer or water! I never feel bloated from beer, I'm never hungover (ha!), and I have just as much fun when I'm with my friends even though I'm not drinking. Of course I'll probably have a glass of wine every now and again with dinner (or champagne at my wedding), but to go back to partying like I used to—I think I'm over that. I am so thankful that Cinch! has taught me the right way to eat.

It was also really great that my friend Miri and I did this together. Having that support was amazing. We would talk about our meals, eat lunch together, and get excited about each other's results. Even when I went away for the weekend, I was able to stick with the plan. I preplanned my meals and snacks and loaded up on Lärabars and the portable snacks Cynthia recommends. I can't believe it was this easy!

I'm absolutely thrilled with my results. I'm so excited and I've been telling everyone! I am going to continue the Cinch! program and I am looking forward to my new lifestyle.

---

## storing herbs and spices

Many seasonings start to lose their potency about six months after being opened, so buy small amounts and use them up. To remind yourself when you purchased them, tape a small sticky note to each container and write in the date. Dried herbs and spices should be stocked in airtight containers in your cupboard. Heat, humidity, and excessive light will cause them to lose their favor more quickly.

If you buy fresh herbs and have extra, you can chop and freeze them in ice-cube trays. Here's the trick: fill the tray just half way up with water. Add the chopped herbs, and freeze about thirty minutes. After the half cubes are semifrozen, add water to fill the tray completely. This will suspend the herbs in the center of each cube. Otherwise, they'll float to the top and be susceptible to freezer burn. When you need an herb, just melt a cube or two.

---

To save time when I cook, I sometimes buy preminced garlic cloves jarred in water. But whenever possible, I use fresh garlic. Look for firm bulbs free from soft spots or sprouts, and store garlic uncovered or loosely covered at room temperature in a cool, dry spot, where it will keep for a few months. Garlic will get too moist in the fridge.

A Tufts University study published in the *Journal of Nutrition* found that adding turmeric to your diet could stall weight gain by preventing new blood-vessel growth—a process called angiogenesis, which is needed to build fat tissue. In the study, different mice were assigned for twelve weeks to a low-fat diet or a high-fat diet; within each group, some subjects also ingested curcumin—the potent antioxidant that gives turmeric its bright color. Even on a high-fat diet, the curcumin group gained less body fat, even without a reduced food intake. They also had less blood-vessel growth in their fat tissue and lower levels of blood sugar, triglycerides, cholesterol, and liver fat.

## ready, set, season!

Using these seasonings in every meal will help curb your appetite, and they contain natural properties that can speed up weight loss. The Cinch! plan maximizes these amazing benefits because SASS is the "secret weapon" in every meal. You'll quickly get into the habit of using one or more of these five delicious categories of health-promoting seasonings every time you eat. So by the end of thirty days, a dash of cinnamon, teaspoon of fresh garlic, or dose of citrus juice will replace your usual sugary and salty sauces and additives. The SASS seasonings will also open up a whole new world of flavor, so you'll look forward to every meal and see results without ever feeling deprived and never feeling like you're eating "diet" food. Rather than plain yogurt with fruit, boring air-popped popcorn, and bland chicken, you'll enjoy the Pineapple Peppercorn Almond Parfait, Cranberry Parmesan Herbed Popcorn, and Chicken Satay Pita. As I've discovered, SASS is the key to helping you achieve weight loss while savoring every morsel of your meals.

# 4

24 25 26 27 28 29 30 31 32 33

# the cinch! core

H ere's the ultimate weight-loss plan you've been waiting for! This chapter includes all you need to know to master Cinch! Get ready to eat real food, not diet stuff. With this plan, each meal is like a feast for your senses, and you'll see quick results without feeling the least bit hungry or deprived. It's also incredibly easy to follow. The plan is literally as simple as a five-piece puzzle, and once you have it down, you can follow it anytime, anywhere, whether you're at home, at a restaurant, or on vacation.

The foundation of Cinch! is the five-piece puzzle. Each meal is constructed from five pieces: (1) produce; (2) a whole grain; (3) lean protein; (4) plant-based fat; and (5) SASS. Breakfast and snack options contain fruit; lunch and dinner contain veggies. Otherwise, the configuration of all the meals is identical.

I have chosen this configuration because I believe it provides the best ratio of carbs, protein, and fat for weight loss, blood-sugar control, and satiety, as well as the broad spectrum of nutrients and antioxidants that you need to look and feel your best and protect your health.

This consistent, "fixed" meal structure ensures that you'll eat the precise foods and portions needed to shed excess pounds while feeling fantastic every step of the way. That's because you'll be eating such clean, nutrient-rich food that you'll be assured of an optimal intake of all the right stuff—vitamins, minerals, antioxidants, fiber, lean protein, and good carbs and fat. Without even realizing it, you'll eat the perfect portions and number of servings from each food group each day. That means you'll never end a day without fitting in at least two servings of fruit and four veggies and the recommended minimum three servings of whole grains. You also won't miss out on protein or good-for-you fats, because they're built into every breakfast, lunch, dinner, and snack.

I've already done the work for you. Each meal in this chapter contains all five pieces of the puzzle in the right amounts and tells you exactly how to assemble the meals. Each day, your foolproof plan is ready for you. All you need to do is:

> 24 25 26 27 28 29 30
>
> I woke up hungry! That never happens, and the first thought that went through my head was how delicious breakfast will be.
>
> AMANDA, AGE 22

1. Look through the meal lists.
2. Choose any breakfast, lunch, dinner, and snack meal you like; you can repeat individual meals as often as you like.
3. Make the meals exactly as stated.
4. Stick to the eating schedule.

Once you've decided which meals to prepare and have shopped for the ingredients, you'll have everything you need to follow through. If you need more support, including videos of a Cinch! grocery tour and cooking demonstrations, visit me at www.cinchyourself.com. For more tips about planning ahead and how to use the five-piece puzzle to construct new meals on your own, see chapter 6.

## how to make smart substitutions

To maintain the proper balance of nutrients, it's important to make the meals exactly as they're written. However, if there is an ingredient you don't have or don't like, you can make a substitution. Just make sure to swap out only foods within the same food group. In other words, if you loathe onions, you can omit them and use the same amount of another veggie, like mushrooms, but you can't exchange onions for more of an ingredient from a different food group, such as barley, beans, or nuts. For lists that lay out which foods fall into which groups, see chapter 6.

## beverages

Allowed beverages include:

- Water, iced or hot; minimum of eight cups, maximum of two and a half liters (ten cups).
- All-natural, calorie-free seltzer. The only ingredients you should see on the can or bottle are carbonated water and natural flavoring. Count seltzer toward your total water intake.
- All-natural, calorie-free, flavored flat water (no bubbles). The only ingredients you should see are water and natural flavoring. Count flat water toward your total water intake.
- Freshly brewed iced or hot black, oolong, green, white, red, or herbal tea, unsweetened; maximum of five cups per day.
- Bottled unsweetened brewed iced tea, flat or sparkling. Count toward your total tea intake.
- Coffee; limit of one cup (eight ounces) per day, with maximum of one-quarter cup organic skim or organic soy milk, no artificial

sweeteners; add one teaspoon or one packet raw sugar if desired, and flavor with spices such as cinnamon, nutmeg, or cloves. Soy milks labeled vanilla or plain generally have about the equivalent of two cubes of sugar added per cup. If you use these flavors, as opposed to unsweetened soy milk, don't add the packet of raw sugar. (If you're not a coffee drinker, you can skip this, but you don't get to add an additional cup of tea to compensate.)

- Zesty Cinnamon Basil Berry Tea, maximum of one recipe per day. (See page 21 for the recipe.)

## cinch! meals

The meals are listed based on the foods they include, as follows.

- Dairy meals include dairy and plant-based foods.
- Egg meals include eggs and plant-based foods.
- Vegan meals contain only plant-based foods.
- Chicken meals include chicken and plant-based foods.
- Turkey meals include turkey and plant-based foods.
- Seafood meals include seafood and plant-based foods.

If you're an omnivore (you eat all animal-based foods), you have an additional rule: choose at least five vegetarian or vegan meals per week. If you're a vegetarian, choose at least five vegan meals per week. In chapter 7 I explain why this strategy will significantly boost your results.

## why red meat isn't included

Yes, you can lose weight on a diet that includes red meat. But for numerous reasons, I do not recommend it, and I have not included beef or pork in the Cinch! meals.

I've long been a fan of a Mediterranean style of eating, which I consider to be the gold standard for health and disease prevention. In Mediterranean countries, where people live long, healthy lives and rates of heart disease are much lower than ours, red meat is rarely consumed. In countless published studies, people who regularly eat red meat have higher rates of cancer, heart disease, and overall mortality.

A recent British study found that women with the highest intake of red meat, the equivalent to one portion a day, had a 56 percent greater risk of developing breast cancer than those who ate none. Researchers from the National Cancer Institute (NCI) report that high intakes of red and processed meats may raise the risk of lung and colorectal cancer by up to 20 percent and may increase the risk of prostate cancer by 12 percent and of advanced prostate cancer by 30 percent.

When NCI scientists studied the diets and disease rates of more than five hundred thousand middle-aged adults over ten years, they found that the men and women who ate the most red meat (averaging two ounces per 1,000 calories per day) had a higher risk for overall death, death from heart disease, and death from cancer than those who ate the least red meat (an average of one-third of an ounce per 1,000 calories per day). The same results applied to the consumption of processed meats such as salami, bologna, and roast beef.

Meat also is a major source of saturated fat, which has been associated with breast and colorectal cancer. Finally, lower red-meat intakes have been tied to lower levels of blood pressure and cholesterol—two major risk factors for heart disease, the nation's number one killer.

What's more, in the United States, red meat has been the source of several recent food-safety scares. In 2009, over 800,000 pounds of ground beef were recalled after an outbreak of antibiotic-resistant salmonella that sickened people across nine states. The same year, nearly 546,000 pounds of ground beef sold in New York and at least seven other states were re-called after evidence of a possible *E. coli* outbreak and at least two deaths.

Hamburgers and sirloin steaks may be tasty, but in my opinion, red meat is not worth the risk.

The Mediterranean style of eating you're following in this plan em-phasizes in-season fruits and vegetables, whole grains, plant-based fats, and, if desired, small amounts of animal protein, preferably from organi-cally raised animals. One reason the Mediterranean diet has remained the key to health and longevity for so many decades is that it has resisted the modernization of our food supply, including the greater influx of animal products, sugary drinks, and processed foods.

I call my plan a "retrotarian" diet. It simply includes back-to-basics meals made from whole foods and seasoned with natural ingredients. Each meal in this chapter makes one serving and contains all five pieces of the puzzle in the right amounts.

## the five puzzle pieces

Rather than listing each meal's ingredients in traditional recipe format, which lists them in the order in which they are presented in the recipe instructions, I did something different. You'll always see the ingredients listed according to the five puzzle pieces in the same order:

Produce (fruit in the breakfast and snack meals, veggies in the lunch and dinner meals)
Whole grain
Lean protein
Plant-based fat
SASS

Consistently seeing each meal's ingredients this way helps the "puzzle principle" become second nature. As you read through each recipe, you will easily see which ingredients fill each piece of the puzzle. Here's an example of one of my favorite meals in the plan:

## Black Bean Tacos with Cilantro-Jalapeño Guacamole

*Produce:* 1 cup fresh mushrooms, chopped; ½ cup each fresh spinach and onions (any type), diced; ¼ cup low-sodium vegetable broth
*Whole grain:* 2 soft taco-size whole-corn tortillas
*Lean protein:* ½ cup black beans
*Plant-based fat:* ¼ of a medium avocado, mashed
*SASS:* Dash freshly ground cracked black pepper; 1 teaspoon fresh, chopped cilantro; 1 small jalapeño, diced; and wedges of fresh lime

Mix pepper, cilantro, and jalapeño into avocado and chill. On the stove top over medium heat, sauté vegetables in broth until tender. Warm tortillas, fill with beans and vegetables (serve extra vegetables on side), and garnish with fresh lime and top with avocado.

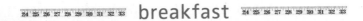 breakfast

## dairy meals

## Blueberry Smoothie with Almond Toast

*Produce:* 1 cup frozen blueberries
*Whole grain:* 1 slice whole-grain bread
*Lean protein:* 8 ounces organic skim milk
*Plant-based fat:* 2 tablespoons natural almond butter
*SASS:* Pinch ground nutmeg

Toast the bread, and spread with the almond butter. Serve with a smoothie made by whipping together the berries, milk, and nutmeg in a blender.

## Chocolate Pear Ginger Smoothie

*Produce:* **1 small pear, sliced**
*Whole grain:* **¼ cup whole oats**
*Lean protein:* **8 ounces organic skim milk**
*Plant-based fat:* **¼ cup chocolate chips**
*SASS:* **½ teaspoon freshly grated ginger**

Place the pear slices, oats, milk, chocolate chips, and ginger in a blender, and whip until smooth.

## Strawberry Cardamom Smoothie with Cashew Oatmeal

*Produce:* **1 cup frozen strawberries**
*Whole grain:* **¼ cup dry whole oats**
*Lean protein:* **8 ounces organic skim milk**
*Plant-based fat:* **2 tablespoons natural cashew butter**
*SASS:* **Pinch cardamom**

Cook the oats with water, and then swirl in the cashew butter. Whip the berries, milk, and cardamom in a blender until smooth.

## Mulberry Almond Parfait

*Produce:* **¼ cup unsweetened dried mulberries**
*Whole grain:* **1 serving cold whole-grain cereal
(see package for serving size)**
*Lean protein:* **6 ounces plain nonfat organic yogurt**
*Plant-based fat:* **2 tablespoons sliced almonds**
*SASS:* **Pinch ground cloves**

Lightly dust the yogurt with the ground cloves and stir. Layer in a dish, alternating with the cereal, mulberries, and almonds.

## Zesty Cranberry Walnut Parfait

*Produce:* **¼ cup dried cranberries sweetened
with fruit juice**
*Whole grain:* **¼ cup whole oats**
*Lean protein:* **6 ounces plain nonfat organic yogurt**

*Plant-based fat:* **2 tablespoons whole walnuts, chopped**

*SASS:* **¼ teaspoon orange zest**

Stir the orange zest into the yogurt. Layer in a dish, alternating with the oats, cranberries, and walnuts.

## Spicy Grape Parfait

*Produce:* **1 cup fresh red, white, or black seedless grapes, sliced in half**

*Whole grain:* **1 serving cold whole-grain cereal (see package for serving size)**

*Lean protein:* **6 ounces plain nonfat organic yogurt**

*Plant-based fat:* **2 tablespoons sunflower seeds**

*SASS:* **Dash each ground cinnamon, ground cloves, and freshly ground cracked black pepper**

Stir the spices into the yogurt. Layer in a dish, alternating with the cereal, grapes, and sunflower seeds.

## Banana Hazelnut Ricotta Toast

*Produce:* **1 mini (five-inch) banana, sliced**

*Whole grain:* **1 slice whole-grain bread**

*Lean protein:* **¼ cup nonfat organic ricotta cheese**

*Plant-based fat:* **2 tablespoons whole hazelnuts, chopped**

*SASS:* **Pinch ground cloves**

Stir the cloves into the ricotta. Toast the bread. Spread with the ricotta and top with the hazelnuts and then the banana slices.

## Black Currant Crunch

*Produce:* **¼ cup unsweetened, or fruit-juice-sweetened, dried black currants**

*Whole grain:* **½ whole-grain English muffin**

*Lean protein:* **1 Gouda mini Babybel**

*Plant-based fat:* **2 tablespoons slivered almonds**

*SASS:* **Pinch freshly ground cracked pepper**

Toast the English muffin half. Spread with the Gouda and dust with the pepper. Top with the currants and almonds.

## Strawberry Green Tea Muesli

*Produce:* **1 cup strawberries**
*Whole grain:* **1 serving cold whole-grain cereal (see package for serving size)**
*Lean protein:* **6 ounces plain nonfat organic yogurt**
*Plant-based fat:* **2 tablespoons whole peanuts, chopped**
*SASS:* **½ teaspoon green-tea leaves and 1 small fresh vanilla bean or 1 teaspoon pure vanilla extract**

Stir the vanilla extract or contents from inside bean and the green-tea leaves into the yogurt. Fold in the berries, cereal, and nuts.

## Raspberry Brazil Nut Pita

*Produce:* **1 cup raspberries, fresh, or frozen and thawed**
*Whole grain:* **½ whole-grain pita**
*Lean protein:* **½ cup nonfat organic cottage cheese**
*Plant-based fat:* **2 tablespoons whole Brazil nuts, chopped or crushed**
*SASS:* **Pinch ground nutmeg**

Fold the nutmeg, berries, and nuts into the cottage cheese, and fill the pita with the mixture.

# egg meals

## Berry Almond French Toast

*Produce:* **1 cup raspberries, fresh, or frozen and thawed**
*Whole grain:* **1 slice whole-grain bread**
*Lean protein:* **¼ cup organic egg whites, 1 whole organic egg, or whites from 3 large organic eggs**
*Plant-based fat:* **2 tablespoons slivered almonds**
*SASS:* **Dash each ground cinnamon, ground nutmeg, and ground cloves**

Soak the bread in the eggs. Spray a pan with nonstick cooking spray. Place the soaked bread into the pan, pour excess egg over top of bread, and cook on the stove top, flipping until each side is golden brown. Transfer the bread to a plate, dust with the spices, and top with the berries and almonds.

## Breakfast Tacos with Fresh Figs

*Produce:* **3 medium fresh figs, sliced**

*Whole grain:* **2 soft taco-size whole-corn tortillas**

*Lean protein:* **¼ cup organic egg whites, 1 whole organic egg, or whites from 3 large organic eggs**

*Plant-based fat:* **¼ medium avocado, mashed**

*SASS:* **Dash freshly ground cracked black pepper; 1 teaspoon fresh, chopped cilantro; and 1 small jalapeño, diced**

Mix the black pepper, cilantro, and jalapeño into the avocado, and chill. Scramble the eggs, using a nonstick spray. Warm the tortillas, fill with the scrambled eggs, and top with the avocado mixture. Serve with the sliced figs.

## Pesto Breakfast Pita

*Produce:* **1 cup fresh red, black, or green grapes**

*Whole grain:* **½ whole-grain pita**

*Lean protein:* **¼ cup organic egg whites, 1 whole organic egg, or whites from 3 large organic eggs**

*Plant-based fat:* **1 tablespoon jarred basil pesto**

*SASS:* **Dash cracked black pepper**

Whisk the pepper into the eggs and scramble, using a nonstick spray. Spread the inside of the pita with the pesto, fill with the scrambled eggs, and serve with a side of grapes.

## Cranberry Walnut Quinoa Pilaf

*Produce:* **¼ cup fruit-juice-sweetened dried cranberries**

*Whole grain:* **½ cup cooked quinoa**

*Lean protein:* **¼ cup organic egg whites, 1 whole organic egg, or whites from 3 large organic eggs**

*Plant-based fat:* **2 tablespoons walnuts, chopped**

*SASS:* **1 teaspoon fresh or ½ teaspoon dried rosemary, and dash cracked black pepper**

Whisk the rosemary and pepper into the eggs. Add the cranberries and walnuts, and scramble, using a nonstick cooking spray. Serve over a bed of warm quinoa.

## Very Berry Omelet with Avocado Toast

*Produce:* 1 cup mixed berries, fresh, or frozen and thawed

*Whole grain:* 1 slice whole-grain bread

*Lean protein:* ¼ cup organic egg whites, 1 whole organic egg, or whites from 3 large organic eggs

*Plant-based fat:* ¼ medium avocado, mashed

*SASS:* Dash each cinnamon, nutmeg, and cloves; and 3 or 4 fresh mint leaves, chopped

Whisk the spices into the eggs. Add the berries and cook on the stove top, using a nonstick cooking spray. Gently fold continuously until the eggs are no longer runny. Transfer to a plate and garnish with the mint. Toast the bread, and spread with the mashed avocado.

## vegan meals

## Dark Chocolate Oatmeal with a Side of Minted Blueberry Yogurt

*Produce:* 1 cup blueberries, fresh, or frozen and thawed

*Whole grain:* ¼ cup dry whole oats, cooked with water

*Lean protein:* 6 ounces coconut or organic soy yogurt

*Plant-based fat:* ¼ cup chocolate chips

*SASS:* 3 or 4 fresh mint leaves, chopped

Stir the chocolate chips into the cooked oats. Fold the blueberries and mint into the yogurt, and serve as a side dish.

## Pear Ginger Almond Pancakes

*Produce:* 1 small pear, sliced

*Whole grain:* 1/3 cup all-natural buckwheat pancake mix

*Lean protein:* 8 ounces nondairy "milk"

*Plant-based fat:* 2 tablespoons sliced almonds

*SASS:* ½ teaspoon fresh grated ginger and 1 tablespoon lemon juice mixed with 1 tablespoon water

Toss the pear slices with the lemon-water mixture and ginger, and microwave for four minutes. Stir 2 tablespoons water into the pancake mix. Cook pancakes on the stove top until golden, and transfer them to a plate. Top first with the pear-ginger mixture and then the almonds, and serve with a side of chilled "milk."

## Raspberry Pistachio Cereal

*Produce:* 1 cup raspberries, fresh, or frozen and thawed
*Whole grain:* 1 serving cold whole-grain cereal (see package for serving size)
*Lean protein:* 8 ounces nondairy "milk"
*Plant-based fat:* 2 tablespoons shelled, unsalted pistachios
*SASS:* Pinch ground cloves

Add the cereal and "milk" to a bowl, lightly dust with the ground cloves, and top with the raspberries and pistachios.

## Peanut Butter Blackberry Toast

*Produce:* 1 cup blackberries, fresh, or frozen and thawed
*Whole grain:* 1 slice whole-grain bread
*Lean protein:* 8 ounces nondairy "milk"
*Plant-based fat:* 2 tablespoons natural peanut butter
*SASS:* Pinch ground nutmeg

Toast the bread and spread it with the peanut butter. Top with the blackberries, lightly dust with the nutmeg, and serve with a chilled side of "milk."

## California Harvest Pita with Minted Yogurt

*Produce:* 1 cup red, black, or green seedless grapes
*Whole grain:* ½ whole-grain pita
*Lean protein:* 6 ounces nondairy "yogurt"
*Plant-based fat:* 2 tablespoons cashew butter
*SASS:* 3 or 4 fresh mint leaves, chopped

Slice the grapes in half. Spread the inside of the pita with the cashew butter, and fill with the grapes. Serve with a side of yogurt mixed with the fresh, chopped mint.

## Strawberry Avocado Tacos

*Produce:* 1 cup strawberries, fresh, or frozen and thawed, sliced
*Whole grain:* 2 soft taco-size whole-corn tortillas
*Lean protein:* ½ cup shelled organic edamame, fresh, or frozen and thawed, or ⅕ of a 14-ounce package of extra-firm organic tofu, crumbled

*Plant-based fat:* ¼ medium avocado, chopped
*SASS:* 1 tablespoon each balsamic vinegar and fresh, chopped oregano

Mix the sliced strawberries with the edamame or tofu, avocado, and oregano. Drizzle with the balsamic vinegar, and fill the tortillas with the strawberry mixture.

## Apple Pecan Breakfast Pilaf

*Produce:* 1 small apple with skin, shredded
*Whole grain:* ½ cup cooked, chilled brown rice
*Lean protein:* 1 cup coconut milk
*Plant-based fat:* 2 tablespoons whole pecans, chopped
*SASS:* Pinch ground cinnamon

Mix the cooked, chilled brown rice with the coconut milk, cinnamon, and apple, and top with the chopped pecans.

## Cranberry Cashew Parfait

*Produce:* ¼ cup dried cranberries sweetened with fruit juice
*Whole grain:* 1 serving puffed whole-grain cereal (see package for serving size), no sugar added
*Lean protein:* 6 ounces nondairy "yogurt"
*Plant-based fat:* 2 tablespoons whole cashews, chopped
*SASS:* Pinch ground cloves

Mix the cranberries, cereal, and cashews into the yogurt, and lightly dust with the cloves.

## Green Tea and Vanilla Banana Almond Smoothie

*Produce:* 1 mini (five-inch) banana or ½ cup frozen sliced banana
*Whole grain:* ¼ cup whole oats
*Lean protein:* 8 ounces nondairy "milk"
*Plant-based fat:* 2 tablespoons natural almond butter
*SASS:* ½ teaspoon green-tea leaves and 1 small fresh vanilla bean or 1 teaspoon pure vanilla extract

In a blender, whip together the banana, oats, "milk," almond butter, green tea, and vanilla extract or contents from inside bean until smooth. Pour the mixture into a glass and serve.

## Peanut Butter Mulberry Toast

*Produce:* **¼ cup unsweetened dried mulberries**
*Whole grain:* **1 slice whole-grain bread**
*Lean protein:* **8 ounces nondairy "milk"**
*Plant-based fat:* **2 tablespoons natural peanut butter**
*SASS:* **Pinch ground nutmeg**

Toast the bread and spread it with the peanut butter. Sprinkle with the nutmeg, top with the mulberries, and serve with a side of chilled "milk."

## Cherry Almond Green Tea Smoothie

*Produce:* **1 cup frozen pitted cherries**
*Whole grain:* **¼ cup whole oats**
*Lean protein:* **8 ounces nondairy "milk"**
*Plant-based fat:* **2 tablespoons natural almond butter**
*SASS:* **1 teaspoon green-tea leaves and pinch ground cinnamon**

In a blender, whip together the cherries, oats, "milk," almond butter, tea leaves, and cinnamon until smooth. Pour the mixture into a glass and serve.

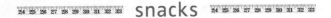

## snacks

## dairy meals

## Peppery Kiwi Almond Crunch

*Produce:* **1 medium kiwi, peeled and sliced**
*Whole grain:* **1 slice whole-grain bread**
*Lean protein:* **¼ cup nonfat organic ricotta cheese**
*Plant-based fat:* **2 tablespoons sliced almonds**
*SASS:* **3 twists cracked black peppercorns**

Fold the pepper into the ricotta. Toast the bread, spread with the ricotta, and top with the almonds and then the kiwi slices.

## grapes, the secret berry

When you look over the two daily meals that include fruit—breakfast and snack—you'll notice that one category of fruits occurs more frequently than any other: berries. When most people think of berries, raspberries, blueberries, and strawberries come to mind, but did you know that grapes are also a member of the berry family?

Technically, these beauties are small round or oval berries that grow on woody vines. The botanical definition of a berry is a simple fruit produced from a single ovary, part of the female reproductive organ of flowering plants, and that's just what grapes are.

Grapes originated in what is now southern Turkey and were a staple in the diet of ancient Greeks and Romans. Grapes grow in clusters of six to three hundred berries. There are dozens of varieties, and they can be red, black, dark blue, yellow, green, pink, and even "white" (actually light green).

Grapes are a particularly potent source of antioxidants called *flavonoids*. Generally, the richer the color, the higher the concentration of flavonoids. Two flavonoids in particular, quercitin and resveratrol, have been shown to decrease the risk of heart disease by relaxing blood vessels to open up blood flow, preventing blood clots and protecting "bad" LDL cholesterol from becoming oxidized.

In a nutshell, oxidation is caused by nasty substances called free radicals, which build up in our body as a normal part of metabolism, and build up even more when we're under stress. Free radicals are oxygen molecules that have become unstable (think of a chair with three legs). In an attempt to balance themselves, they attack the DNA in healthy cells. When LDL cholesterol gets oxidized or attacked by free radicals, it becomes more dangerous, triggering a domino effect that leads to inflammation, harder arteries, and blockages.

Antioxidants like the ones found in grapes fight this. A study from Northeastern Ohio Universities Colleges of Medicine also found that resveratrol directly affects heart-muscle cells, keeping them healthy. A study published in *Cancer Research* showed that red-grape skins help reduce the size of estrogen-dependent breast-cancer tumors, and this berry's resveratrol has been linked to a reduction in the brain plaques associated with Alzheimer's disease.

I'm a huge fan of all berries, and I love spreading the word that grapes are a member of the family. To reap the benefits, aim for at least three berry-based breakfasts or snack meals per week.

## Mango Mint Avocado Smoothie

*Produce:* **1 cup fresh mango, chopped, or frozen chopped mango**
*Whole grain:* **¼ cup whole oats**
*Lean protein:* **8 ounces organic skim milk**
*Plant-based fat:* **¼ medium avocado**
*SASS:* **1 tablespoon each fresh lime juice
and chopped fresh mint**

In a blender, whip all the ingredients until smooth.

## Sonoma Snack

*Produce:* **1 cup red seedless grapes**
*Whole grain:* **1 serving all-natural whole-grain crackers
(see package for serving size)**
*Lean protein:* **1 mini Babybel spreadable cheese**
*Plant-based fat:* **10 whole black olives**
*SASS:* **1 teaspoon fresh or ½ teaspoon dried rosemary**

Spread the cheese on crackers, and garnish with the rosemary. Serve with the grapes and olives.

## Tangerine Almond Twist

*Produce:* **Wedges from 1 medium tangerine,
seeds removed, chopped**
*Whole grain:* **½ whole-grain pita**
*Lean protein:* **½ cup nonfat organic cottage cheese**
*Plant-based fat:* **2 tablespoons sliced almonds**
*SASS:* **½ teaspoon tangerine zest
and 3 or 4 fresh basil leaves, chopped**

Fold the tangerine zest and basil into the **cottage** cheese, and then mix in the chopped tangerine wedges. Fill the pita with the tangerine mixture, and garnish with the almonds.

## Cranberry Parmesan Herbed Popcorn

*Produce:* ¼ cup dried cranberries sweetened with fruit juice
*Whole grain:* ¼ cup unpopped popcorn kernels
*Lean protein:* ¼ cup shredded Parmesan
*Plant-based fat:* 1 tablespoon high-oleic sunflower oil
*SASS:* 1 teaspoon Italian herb seasoning mix

Place the popcorn kernels and oil in a heavy pan, cover, and shake over medium heat until popped. Mix in the cranberries, and then sprinkle with the Parmesan and herbs.

## Cinnamon Walnut Apple Crisp

*Produce:* 1 medium apple with skin, finely chopped
*Whole grain:* ¼ cup whole oats
*Lean protein:* 8 ounces organic skim milk
*Plant-based fat:* 2 tablespoons walnuts, chopped
*SASS:* 1 tablespoon lemon juice and $^1/_8$ teaspoon cinnamon

Toss the chopped apple with the lemon juice and cinnamon, and microwave on high for five minutes. Top with the oats and walnuts, and serve with a side of milk.

## Broiled Grapefruit with Herbed Feta

*Produce:* 1 small grapefruit
*Whole grain:* 1 serving all-natural whole-grain crackers
(see package for serving size)
*Lean protein:* ¼ cup reduced-fat organic feta cheese
*Plant-based fat:* 2 tablespoons whole chestnuts, chopped
*SASS:* 1 teaspoon fresh or ½ teaspoon dried dill
and 1 teaspoon fresh or ½ teaspoon dried parsley

Preheat the broiler.
Mix the herbs and chestnuts into the feta. Halve the grapefruit, and heat the halves under the broiler for about three to five minutes. Top with the feta, and serve with the crackers.

# MY STORY

### Miri Frankel, 30 | Pounds lost: 11.25

## I Lost 10.5 Inches Including 5 from My Waist!

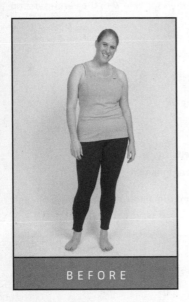

BEFORE

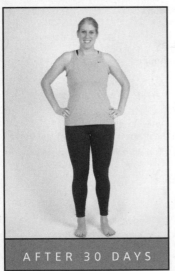

AFTER 30 DAYS

My friend and co-worker Heidi was getting married at the end of August, so when she saw an invitation to try out a weight-loss plan, she jumped on it. When she asked me if I wanted to do it with her I decided to go for it, and now I owe her one heck of a wedding present!

I'm a runner so I was very muscular and fit, but despite all of my training I was carrying extra body fat. Cinch! was exactly what I needed. I was always mindful of eating a balanced diet rather than "dieting," especially given my running schedule. But my real ah-ha moment was learning that my perspective of a balanced diet was off in my proportions. Changing those proportions finally made those stubborn pounds and inches come off!

The first day I thought I ate too much food because I ate so well and didn't feel too hungry between meals. I actually went back to review the plan to make sure I didn't overdo anything, but I knew I used the right amounts because I measured.

On the second day for lunch I had the Smoked Gouda and Grilled Onion Salad. It was so delicious I knew I could follow this plan for the next twenty-eight days! Um, the oatmeal was like dessert, so decadent....I thought, this can't be a diet. ☺ What a fun breakfast!

And within the first week my tight jeans that I didn't wear very often weren't so tight.

It was such a great experience to learn that I can eat the healthy, balanced foods I love in a way that keeps the scale going down... down... down. I'm also eating more variety. I used to stick to the same couple of quick prep meals, but I found out that it's easier than I thought to cook a wide variety of interesting healthy meals at home. And I can still have my favorite foods like pasta; I just have to balance them.

I love making up my own Cinch! meals and having the flexibility to "play with my food" based on the ingredients I have on hand. I can make meals influenced by my cravings and mood, like pizza one day, pasta the next. Everything is hearty and filling and Cinch! combinations are ones I wouldn't have thought to put together myself. For example, the Cranberry Pesto Egg Spread snack is *really* delicious!

I am an anti-calorie-counter. If I have to track calories or points all day or week, I'll never stick with it. Learning to balance my diet using the Cinch! method was easy, and because it makes me feel and look good, it's a real (and realistic) lifestyle, not a go-on, go-off diet.

I am beyond excited about my results, and all my friends and family are so proud of my results. I always knew those last stubborn pounds and untoned body parts were probably due to nutrition rather than exercise. This experience showed me I was right—and how to change that!

It makes me feel so great to see how much better I look and how much better I feel! I think I probably have about five more pounds to lose to really get rid of the stubborn flabby bits. I'm happy that I can do it with a safe, healthy, and satisfying eating plan!

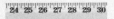

## Peppery Pear Crunch

> I can eat like this for the rest of my life.
>
> CHRIS, AGE 54

*Produce:* **1 medium pear, sliced**
*Whole grain:* **½ whole-grain English muffin**
*Lean protein:* **1 mini Babybel Gouda**
*Plant-based fat:* **2 tablespoons slivered almonds**
*SASS:* **3 twists cracked black peppercorns**

Toast the English muffin half. Spread with the Gouda, and dust with the pepper. Top with the pear slices and almonds.

## Strawberry Vanilla Hazelnut "Ice Cream"

*Produce:* **1 cup strawberries, fresh, or frozen and thawed, sliced**
*Whole grain:* **¼ cup whole oats**
*Lean protein:* **6 ounces nonfat plain organic yogurt**
*Plant-based fat:* **2 tablespoons whole hazelnuts, chopped**
*SASS:* **1 small fresh vanilla bean or 1 teaspoon pure vanilla extract**

Fold the vanilla extract or contents from inside bean into the yogurt. Add the strawberries, oats, and hazelnuts. Place in a sealable container and freeze for at least thirty minutes. Eat with a spoon, like ice cream.

## Pineapple Avocado Tacos

*Produce:* **1 cup fresh sliced pineapple or ½ cup canned in natural juice**
*Whole grain:* **2 soft taco-size whole-corn tortillas**
*Lean protein:* **¼ cup reduced-fat organic feta cheese**
*Plant-based fat:* **¼ medium avocado**
*SASS:* **Dash freshly ground cracked black pepper;**
**1 teaspoon fresh chopped cilantro; and 1 small jalapeño, diced**

Mix the pepper, cilantro, and jalapeño into the avocado to make a guacamole, and chill. Warm the tortillas and fill with the pineapple, then the feta, and garnish with the guacamole.

## egg meals

### Open-Faced Pesto Egg Sandwich

*Produce:* **1 cup black seedless grapes**

*Whole grain:* **1 slice whole-grain bread**

*Lean protein:* **1 whole organic hard-boiled egg
or 2 organic hard-boiled egg whites, sliced**

*Plant-based fat:* **1 tablespoon jarred basil pesto**

*SASS:* **1 chili pepper, finely chopped**

Toast the bread. Spread it with the pesto, top with the sliced egg, and garnish with the chopped chili pepper. Serve the grapes on the side.

### Fig and Olive Snack

*Produce:* **3 medium fresh figs**

*Whole grain:* **1 serving all-natural whole-grain crackers
(see package for serving size)**

*Lean protein:* **1 whole organic hard-boiled egg
or 2 organic hard-boiled egg whites**

*Plant-based fat:* **10 green olives**

*SASS:* **1 teaspoon lemon juice and ¹/₈ teaspoon each chopped garlic, chopped
parsley, chopped cilantro, and crushed red pepper**

Toss the olives with the seasonings, and serve with the figs, crackers, and egg.

### Avocado Egg Dip

*Produce:* **1 cup kumquats**

*Whole grain:* **1 serving all-natural whole-grain crackers (see package for
serving size)**

*Lean protein:* **1 whole organic hard-boiled egg or 2 organic hard-boiled egg whites,
chopped**

*Plant-based fat:* **¼ medium avocado, mashed**

*SASS:* **1 teaspoon lemon juice, dash black pepper, and dash cayenne pepper**

Fold the lemon juice and two kinds of pepper into the mashed avocado. Add the chopped egg, and serve with the crackers and kumquats.

## Cranberry Pesto Egg Spread

*Produce:* ¼ cup dried cranberries sweetened with fruit juice

*Whole grain:* 1 serving all-natural whole-grain crackers (see package for serving size)

*Lean protein:* 1 whole organic hard-boiled egg or 2 organic hard-boiled egg whites, chopped

*Plant-based fat:* 1 tablespoon jarred basil pesto

*SASS:* 1 teaspoon fresh or ½ teaspoon dried rosemary

Mix the cranberries, egg, and rosemary into the pesto, and spread on the crackers.

## Spicy Egg Tacos with Cilantro-Jalapeño Guacamole

*Produce:* 1 medium orange

*Whole grain:* 2 soft taco-size whole-corn tortillas

*Lean protein:* 1 whole organic hard-boiled egg or 2 organic hard-boiled egg whites, chopped

*Plant-based fat:* ¼ medium avocado

*SASS:* Dash freshly ground cracked black pepper; 1 teaspoon fresh, chopped cilantro; 1 small jalapeño, diced; and wedges of fresh lime

Mash the pepper, cilantro, and jalapeño into the avocado to make a guacamole, and chill. Warm the tortillas and fill with the chopped egg, top with the guacamole, and garnish with the lime wedges. Serve with the whole orange on the side.

## vegan snacks

## Pineapple Almond Peppercorn Parfait

*Produce:* 1 cup fresh sliced pineapple or ½ cup canned in natural juice

*Whole grain:* ¼ cup dry whole oats

*Lean protein:* 6 ounces coconut or organic soy yogurt

*Plant-based fat:* 2 tablespoons sliced almonds

*SASS:* 3 twists cracked black peppercorn

Fold the pepper into the yogurt. Alternate layers of yogurt, oats, and pineapple in a dish, and garnish with the almonds.

## California Sunshine Salad

*Produce:* Sections from 1 medium orange, seeds removed

*Whole grain:* ½ cup sweet corn, fresh, or frozen and thawed,
or kernels sliced from 1 medium ear of fresh roasted corn, chilled

*Lean protein:* ½ cup chilled organic edamame

*Plant-based fat:* ¼ medium avocado, chopped

*SASS:* 2 tablespoons rice vinegar and ¼ teaspoon each dried thyme,
black pepper, and grated lemon peel

Whisk the vinegar and seasonings together and toss with remaining ingredients.

## Cinch! Picnic Snack

*Produce:* 1 cup cubed cantaloupe

*Whole grain:* 1 serving all-natural whole-grain crackers
(see package for serving size)

*Lean protein:* ⅕ of a 14-ounce package of extra-firm organic tofu,
sliced into cubes

*Plant-based fat:* 1 tablespoon jarred basil pesto

*SASS:* 1 medium jalapeño, minced

Spread the crackers with the pesto, and sprinkle with the minced jalapeño. On toothpicks or wooden skewers, alternate the melon and tofu cubes and serve, with the seasoned crackers on the side.

## Peanut Butter Plum Toast

*Produce:* 1 medium plum, sliced

*Whole grain:* 1 slice whole-grain bread

*Lean protein:* 8 ounces nondairy "milk"

*Plant-based fat:* 2 tablespoons natural peanut butter

*SASS:* Pinch ground nutmeg

Toast the bread and spread with the peanut butter. Top with the plum slices, lightly dust with the nutmeg, and serve with a chilled side of "milk."

## Strawberry Walnut "Ice Cream" with Lime Zest

*Produce:* **1 cup strawberries, fresh, or frozen and thawed, sliced**
*Whole grain:* **¼ cup dry whole oats**
*Lean protein:* **6 ounces nondairy "yogurt"**
*Plant-based fat:* **2 tablespoons walnuts, chopped**
*SASS:* **½ teaspoon fresh lime zest**

Fold the berries, oats, walnuts, and lime zest into the yogurt. Place in a sealable container and freeze for at least 30 minutes. Eat with a spoon, like ice cream.

## Tangerine Tofu Tacos with Cilantro-Jalapeño Guacamole

*Produce:* **Wedges from 1 medium tangerine, seeds removed**
*Whole grain:* **2 soft taco-size whole-corn tortillas**
*Lean protein:* **⅕ of a 14-ounce package of extra-firm organic tofu, crumbled**
*Plant-based fat:* **¼ medium avocado, chopped**
*SASS:* **Dash freshly ground cracked black pepper; 1 teaspoon fresh, chopped cilantro; and 1 small jalapeño, diced**

Mix the pepper, cilantro, and jalapeño into the avocado to make a guacamole, and chill. Warm the tortillas, fill with the tofu and then the tangerine wedges, and serve with the guacamole.

## Herbed Popcorn with a Blueberry Coconut Smoothie

*Produce:* **1 cup blueberries, fresh, or frozen and thawed**
*Whole grain:* **¼ cup unpopped popcorn kernels**
*Lean protein:* **8 ounces nondairy coconut "milk"**
*Plant-based fat:* **1 tablespoon high-oleic sunflower oil**
*SASS:* **1 teaspoon Italian herb seasoning mix**

Place the popcorn kernels and oil in a heavy pan, cover, and shake over medium heat until popped. Sprinkle with the herbs. Whip the berries in a blender together with the coconut "milk" until smooth, and serve with the popcorn.

## Ginger Yogurt with Carambola Crunch

*Produce:* **1 medium carambola (star fruit), seeds removed, finely chopped**
*Whole grain:* **¼ cup whole oats**
*Lean protein:* **6 ounces nondairy "yogurt"**
*Plant-based fat:* **2 tablespoons shelled sunflower seeds**
*SASS:* **½ teaspoon freshly grated ginger**

Fold the grated ginger into the yogurt and transfer to a serving dish. In a small bowl, mix the oats and sunflower seeds with the chopped carambola, and spoon the mixture over the yogurt.

## Cinnamon Cherry Yogurt with Peanut Butter Crackers

*Produce:* **1 cup frozen, thawed pitted cherries**
*Whole grain:* **1 serving all-natural whole-grain crackers (see package for serving size)**
*Lean protein:* **6 ounces nondairy "yogurt"**
*Plant-based fat:* **2 tablespoons natural peanut butter**
*SASS:* **¼ teaspoon cinnamon**

Fold the cinnamon into the yogurt, and add the cherries. Spread the crackers with the peanut butter, and serve with the yogurt.

## Vanilla Almond Frozen Banana

*Produce:* **1 mini (five-inch) banana, peeled but not sliced**
*Whole grain:* **¼ cup whole oats**
*Lean protein:* **6 ounces nondairy "yogurt"**
*Plant-based fat:* **2 tablespoons peanuts, chopped**
*SASS:* **1 small fresh vanilla bean or 1 teaspoon pure vanilla extract**

Mix the peanuts and oats together and set aside. Fold the vanilla extract or contents from inside bean into the yogurt. Dip the banana into the yogurt or spoon the yogurt over the banana to coat it thoroughly. Sprinkle with the nut mixture, wrap in wax paper, and freeze at least twenty minutes.

# why losing weight is like paying off debt

What it takes to lose weight is a little different from what it takes to keep the pounds off. When you're trying to lose, strictness and consistency make a huge difference. But when you're simply trying to maintain, you can enjoy a few splurges here and there and still stay the same size. A "diet" is really a blueprint for eating in a way that will keep you well nourished and get you to your weight goal. It's also a lot like a budget.

Imagine that your income and expenses are fixed and fairly even, so you're basically spending what you're earning. If you splurge on a new sweater or boots every once in a while, you can still stay on budget pretty well. But if you start spending an extra $200 per day every day, week after week, or if you spend an extra $1,000 every weekend, pretty soon your expenses will be much higher than your income and you'll be rapidly building debt. This is similar to overeating and gaining excess body fat. Once you get into a situation like this, you have to make a bigger effort to pay down the debt to get back into balance. When you've been in debt, even an extra $50 per day makes a big difference, because that $50 per day snowballs into $350 a week, $1,500 a month, or $18,250 a year.

In other words, being "over" with your food intake day after day keeps you in debt by a fairly big margin, but sticking to your plan or "budget" can make a big dent in that debt over time. You have to be diligent in the beginning, but you won't have to be so strict forever.

It's true that to maintain a healthy weight you'll always have to be mindful of your budget, but you won't always have to be as careful as I'm asking you to be throughout the next thirty days. So if you feel the urge to sneak an extra tablespoon of almond butter or a handful of berries, think of this analogy and remember: extras right now will mean carrying a heavier debt for a longer time and preventing yourself from quickly getting into the black.

# lunch and dinner

## dairy meals

### Smoked Gouda and Grilled Onion Salad

*Produce:* **1½ cups torn romaine lettuce and
½ cup sliced white or yellow onion**

*Whole grain:* **1 serving all-natural whole-grain crackers
(see package for serving size)**

*Lean protein:* **1 ounce smoked Gouda, diced**

*Plant-based fat:* **1 tablespoon extra-virgin olive oil**

*SASS:* **1 tablespoon balsamic vinegar, 1 teaspoon lemon juice,
and dash cracked black pepper**

On the stove top over medium heat, sauté the sliced onion in the olive oil until translucent. Set aside.

Toss the romaine with the vinegar and lemon juice. Top the lettuce with the sautéed onions, then the Gouda, and dust with the pepper. Serve with crackers.

### Black and Blue Salad

*Produce:* **1 cup field greens and 1 medium vine-ripened tomato,
cut into wedges**

*Whole grain:* **1 serving all-natural whole-grain crackers
(see package for serving size)**

*Lean protein:* **¼ cup crumbled organic blue cheese**

*Plant-based fat:* **10 large black olives, sliced**

*SASS:* **1 tablespoon red wine vinegar
and 1 teaspoon Italian herb seasoning mix**

Toss the field greens with the vinegar and herbs. Transfer to a salad bowl and top with the tomato wedges, then the olives and blue cheese. Serve with crackers.

## Cinch! Caesar Salad

*Produce:* **2 cups torn romaine leaves**
*Whole grain:* **1 serving all-natural whole-grain crackers
(see package for serving size), broken into small pieces**
*Lean protein:* **¼ cup fresh shredded Parmesan**
*Plant-based fat:* **1 tablespoon extra-virgin olive oil**
*SASS:* **1 tablespoon lemon juice and dash cracked black pepper**

Toss the romaine with the olive oil, lemon juice, and pepper. Top with the Parmesan and crackers.

## Ricotta Primavera Penne

*Produce:* **½ cup each chopped mushrooms, chopped onion,
chopped green bell pepper, and chopped vine-ripened or plum tomato**
*Whole grain:* **½ cup cooked whole-grain penne**
*Lean protein:* **¼ cup nonfat organic ricotta cheese**
*Plant-based fat:* **1 tablespoon extra-virgin olive oil**
*SASS:* **½ teaspoon minced garlic and 1 teaspoon Italian herb seasoning mix**

On the stove top over medium heat, sauté the chopped mushrooms, onion, green pepper, and tomato in the olive oil until slightly tender. Mix the ricotta with the garlic and herbs, and toss with pasta. Cover a plate with pasta mixture, and top with the sautéed vegetables.

## Spinach Walnut Feta Pita

*Produce:* **1 cup fresh baby spinach and 1 vine-ripened or plum tomato, diced**
*Whole grain:* **½ whole-grain pita**
*Lean protein:* **¼ cup crumbled organic feta cheese**
*Plant-based fat:* **2 tablespoons walnuts, chopped**
*SASS:* **1 tablespoon balsamic vinegar**

Toss the spinach, tomatoes, feta, and walnuts with the vinegar. Stuff the pita with spinach mixture and serve, with extra veggies on the side.

## Fresh Mozzarella Basil "Pizzalad"

*Produce:* 1 cup field greens and 1 vine-ripened or plum tomato, sliced thin

*Whole grain:* ½ whole-grain pita, sliced widthwise, not lengthwise (slice along edge of round)

*Lean protein:* 1 ounce fresh mozzarella, sliced thin

*Plant-based fat:* 1 tablespoon extra-virgin olive oil

*SASS:* ½ teaspoon minced garlic, 6–8 fresh basil leaves, and 1 tablespoon balsamic vinegar

Lay the pita, outer side facing up, on a piece of foil. Rub the pita with the olive oil. Prebake in the oven at 450°F for three to five minutes or until slightly crisp. Top with the garlic, basil, and mozzarella. Bake in the oven at 450°F for five to eight minutes. Remove from the oven, transfer to a plate, cover with the greens, drizzle with balsamic, and serve.

## Mediterranean Pasta Salad

*Produce:* ½ cup each artichoke hearts (canned or jarred in water, drained and rinsed, or vacuum sealed), fresh baby spinach, diced red pepper, and diced red onion

*Whole grain:* ½ cup cooked whole-grain pasta spirals, chilled

*Lean protein:* ¼ cup crumbled organic feta cheese

*Plant-based fat:* 5 large red and 5 large black olives, sliced

*SASS:* 1 tablespoon red-wine vinegar and 1 teaspoon Italian herb seasoning mix

Toss the pasta with the vinegar, herbs, artichoke hearts, spinach, red pepper, onion, olives, and feta, and serve chilled.

## Spicy Avocado Tostadas

*Produce:* 1 cup chopped romaine, ½ cup minced onion, and ½ cup chopped fresh vine-ripened tomato

*Whole grain:* 2 soft taco-size whole-corn tortillas

*Lean protein:* ¼ cup shredded reduced-fat or part-skim organic Monterey Jack cheese

*Plant-based fat:* ¼ medium avocado, mashed

*SASS:* 1 small jalapeño, minced, and wedges of fresh lime

Lay the tortillas flat and warm them in a toaster oven or under the broiler until slightly crisp. Spread with the mashed avocado, sprinkle with the jalapeño and then the cheese, and cover with the tomato, onion, and romaine. Garnish with the lime wedges.

## Savory Spaghetti Squash with Citrus Zest

*Produce:* **2 cups cooked spaghetti squash**
*Whole grain:* **½ cup cooked wild rice**
*Lean protein:* **1 ounce aged organic Asiago cheese, shredded**
*Plant-based fat:* **1 tablespoon jarred basil pesto**
*SASS:* **½ teaspoon tangerine zest**

Toss the cooked spaghetti squash and wild rice with the pesto to coat. Transfer to a plate. Garnish with the Asiago, and sprinkle with the tangerine zest.

## Herbed Walnut Artichoke Lettuce Wraps

*Produce:* **5 large outer romaine leaves, ½ cup artichoke hearts (canned or jarred in water, drained and rinsed, or vacuum sealed), and ¼ cup each diced onion and minced red bell pepper**
*Whole grain:* **1 serving all-natural whole-grain crackers (see package for serving size), broken into small pieces**
*Lean protein:* **½ cup nonfat organic cottage cheese**
*Plant-based fat:* **2 tablespoons walnuts, chopped**
*SASS:* **Dash cracked black pepper, ½ teaspoon minced garlic, and 1 teaspoon Italian herb seasoning mix**

Fold the pepper, garlic, herbs, artichoke hearts, onion, celery, and walnuts into the cottage cheese. Fill the romaine leaves with cottage cheese mixture, and garnish with the cracker pieces.

## chicken meals

## Green-Tea Chicken with Avocado Corn Salad

*Produce:* **1½ cups field greens or baby romaine, ¼ cup sliced red onion, and ¼ cup jarred all-natural salsa**
*Whole grain:* **½ cup sweet corn, fresh or frozen and thawed, or kernels sliced from 1 medium ear of fresh roasted corn**
*Lean protein:* **3 ounces cooked boneless, skinless chicken breast, diced**
*Plant-based fat:* **¼ medium avocado**
*SASS:* **½ teaspoon green-tea leaves mixed with ⅛ teaspoon each black pepper, garlic powder, and lemon zest**

Mix the tea leaves with the pepper, garlic powder, and lemon zest. Toss the chicken with green-tea mixture, and set aside.

Toss the greens and onion with the salsa to coat. Transfer the greens to a bowl, and top with the corn and then the chicken and avocado.

## Chilled Herbed Chicken Pasta Salad

*Produce:* ½ cup each baby spinach leaves; cherry or grape tomatoes, sliced in half; chopped celery; and chopped red bell pepper

*Whole grain:* ½ cup cooked whole-grain pasta spirals

*Lean protein:* 3 ounces cooked boneless, skinless chicken breast, diced

*Plant-based fat:* 1 tablespoon extra-virgin olive oil

*SASS:* 1 tablespoon balsamic vinegar, and 3 or 4 fresh basil leaves, chopped, or 1 teaspoon Italian herb seasoning mix

Combine all the ingredients in a sealable container. Gently shake to mix and coat thoroughly. Serve chilled.

## Spinach, Artichoke, and Olive Chicken Pasta

*Produce:* ½ cup all-natural marinara sauce, warmed; ½ cup artichoke hearts (canned or jarred in water, drained and rinsed, or vacuum sealed); and 1 cup fresh baby spinach leaves

*Whole grain:* ½ cup cooked whole-grain penne

*Lean protein:* 3 ounces cooked boneless, skinless chicken breast, diced

*Plant-based fat:* 10 large olives, sliced

*SASS:* 3 or 4 fresh basil leaves

Fold the basil, artichoke hearts, and spinach into the warmed marinara, and toss with the penne. Top with the chicken, and garnish with the olives.

## Chicken Pesto Pita

*Produce:* 3 or 4 large romaine leaves, finely chopped; 1 medium plum tomato, diced; and ½ cup finely chopped cucumber

*Whole grain:* ½ whole-grain pita

*Lean protein:* 3 ounces cooked boneless, skinless chicken breast, diced

*Plant-based fat:* 1 tablespoon jarred basil pesto

*SASS:* 2 tablespoons balsamic vinegar and 1 clove roasted garlic

Toss the chicken with pesto and set aside. Toss the romaine, tomato, and cucumber with the vinegar and set aside. Spread the inside of the pita with the roasted garlic. Fill the pita with the chicken and then the tossed vegetables, serving any extra on the side.

## Wild Rice and Chicken Lettuce Wraps
## with Citrus Slaw

*Produce:* 5 or 6 large outer romaine leaves, ¼ cup sliced green onions, and
1 cup shredded purple cabbage

*Whole grain:* ½ cup cooked, chilled wild rice

*Lean protein:* 3 ounces cooked boneless, skinless chicken breast, diced

*Plant-based fat:* 1 tablespoon high-oleic sunflower oil

*SASS:* 1 tablespoon 100 percent pineapple juice, 1 tablespoon rice vinegar,
dash cracked black pepper, 1 tablespoon all-natural Dijon mustard, and
1 teaspoon fresh or ½ teaspoon dried dill

Whisk together the sunflower oil, pineapple juice, vinegar, black pepper, and green
onions. Toss with the cabbage to coat thoroughly to make a slaw. Toss the rice and
chicken with Dijon and dill. Fill the romaine "boats" with the chicken mixture, and
serve with slaw on the side.

## Mediterranean Broccoli Couscous Platter

*Produce:* ¼ cup sliced onion and 1¼ cup broccoli florets

*Whole grain:* ½ cup cooked whole-wheat couscous

*Lean protein:* 3 ounces cooked boneless, skinless chicken breast, diced

*Plant-based fat:* 1 tablespoon extra-virgin olive oil

*SASS:* 1 teaspoon minced garlic

On the stove top over low heat, warm the olive oil. Add the garlic, onions, and broccoli, and sauté until the onions are translucent. Spread couscous over a plate, and
top with the chicken and then the sautéed vegetables.

## Chilled Brown Rice and Vegetable Salad
## with Brazil Nut–Dusted Chicken

*Produce:* 1 cup baby spinach and ¼ cup each sliced white button mushrooms,
sliced green onions, sliced red bell pepper, and sliced tomato

*Whole grain:* ½ cup cooked, cooled wild rice

*Lean protein:* 3 ounces cooked boneless, skinless chicken breast

*Plant-based fat:* 2 tablespoons Brazil nuts, crushed

*SASS:* 3 or 4 fresh basil leaves, chopped, or 1 teaspoon dried basil;
1 tablespoon lemon juice; 2 tablespoons balsamic vinegar; and dash cracked
black pepper

Roll the cooked chicken breast in the crushed Brazil nuts, and set aside. Toss the
chilled rice with the spinach, sliced vegetables, basil, lemon juice, vinegar, and
pepper. Chill the salad, and serve with the chicken.

## Garlicky Barley Vegetable Chicken Soup

*Produce:* ¼ cup each chopped onions, chopped zucchini, chopped carrots, and chopped cauliflower; 1 cup canned Italian tomatoes; and 2 cups low-sodium vegetable or chicken broth

*Whole grain:* ½ cup cooked barley

*Lean protein:* 3 ounces cooked boneless, skinless chicken breast, minced

*Plant-based fat:* 1 tablespoon extra-virgin olive oil

*SASS:* ¼ teaspoon minced garlic and 1 teaspoon Italian seasoning

In a saucepan, sauté the garlic and onion in the oil until the onion is translucent. Add the chopped carrots, zucchini, and cauliflower, and lightly sauté. Add the broth and tomatoes, and bring to a boil. Simmer about five to eight minutes. Stir in the barley, chicken, and herbs to heat through.

## California Chicken Cilantro Burrito Bowl

*Produce:* 3 or 4 romaine leaves, torn; ½ cup all-natural salsa; and ¼ cup each chopped green bell pepper, chopped onion, low-sodium vegetable broth

*Whole grain:* ½ cup cooked brown rice

*Lean protein:* 3 ounces cooked boneless, skinless chicken breast, diced

*Plant-based fat:* ¼ medium avocado

*SASS:* ¼ teaspoon minced garlic and 1 tablespoon chopped cilantro

On the stove top over medium heat, sauté the chopped peppers and onions in the vegetable broth until tender, and set aside. Toss the rice with the garlic and cilantro, and place in the bottom of the salad bowl. Top with the romaine and then the salsa, chicken, and avocado.

## Chicken Satay Pita

*Produce:* 3 or 4 romaine leaves, torn; ¼ cup each chopped celery, chopped onions, chopped red bell pepper, and low-sodium vegetable broth

*Whole grain:* ½ whole-grain pita

*Lean protein:* 3 ounces cooked boneless, skinless chicken breast, diced

*Plant-based fat:* 2 tablespoons natural peanut butter

*SASS:* ¼ teaspoon minced garlic, ⅛ teaspoon freshly grated ginger, and dash crushed red pepper

On the stove top over medium heat, sauté the peppers and onions in the broth until tender, and set aside. Mix the garlic, ginger, and crushed red pepper into the peanut butter, and toss with the diced chicken. Fill the pita with the chicken, sautéed vegetables, chopped celery, and romaine.

## turkey meals

### Turkey Mock Tacos

*Produce:* **4 large outer romaine leaves; ½ cup all-natural salsa; and ¼ cup each chopped red bell pepper, chopped onion, and low-sodium vegetable broth**

*Whole grain:* **½ cup sweet corn, fresh, or frozen and thawed, or kernels sliced from 1 medium ear of fresh roasted corn**

*Lean protein:* **3 ounces cooked extra-lean (99 percent lean) ground turkey**

*Plant-based fat:* **¼ medium avocado, sliced**

*SASS:* **1 tablespoon chopped cilantro and 4 lime wedges**

On the stove top over medium heat, sauté the peppers and onions in the broth until tender, and set aside. Mix the cilantro into the ground turkey. Fill each romaine leaf with corn and turkey, and squeeze fresh lime juice over each filled leaf. Top with the salsa, sautéed vegetables (the broth will have cooked out), and sliced avocado.

### Turkey Pita "Pizzalad"

*Produce:* **½ cup all-natural marinara sauce; ½ cup field greens; ¼ cup each chopped asparagus, chopped red bell pepper, chopped red onion, and shredded carrots**

*Whole grain:* **½ whole-grain pita, sliced widthwise, not lengthwise (slice along edge of round)**

*Lean protein:* **3 ounces cooked extra-lean (99 percent lean) ground turkey**

*Plant-based fat:* **1 tablespoon extra-virgin olive oil**

*SASS:* **½ teaspoon minced garlic and 2 tablespoons balsamic vinegar**

Preheat the oven to 450°F.

Lay pita, outer side facing up, on a piece of foil. Prebake in oven at 450°F for three to five minutes, or until slightly crisp, and remove. Sauté the onion and garlic in the olive oil until the onions are translucent. Add the asparagus, pepper, and carrots, and sauté until tender. Spread the pita with the marinara, and cover with the turkey and sautéed vegetables. Bake at 450°F for five to eight minutes. Remove from the oven and transfer to a plate. Toss the field greens with the vinegar, cover the top of the pita pizza, and serve.

## Turkey Walnut Pita

*Produce:* **1 cup baby spinach, ¼ cup chopped red onion, and 1 plum tomato, diced**

*Whole grain:* **½ whole-grain pita**

*Lean protein:* **3 ounces roasted, baked, or grilled boneless, skinless turkey breast, diced**

*Plant-based fat:* **2 tablespoons walnuts, chopped**

*SASS:* **2 tablespoons balsamic vinegar and dash cracked black pepper**

Place the vegetables, turkey, walnuts, vinegar, and pepper in a small, sealable bowl. Cover, and gently shake to coat. Fill the pita with the turkey mixture.

## Turkey and Wild Rice–Stuffed Peppers

*Produce:* **2 large whole green bell peppers and ¼ cup each minced onion, shredded carrots, baby spinach, and chopped celery**

*Whole grain:* **½ cup cooked wild rice**

*Lean protein:* **3 ounces cooked extra-lean (99 percent lean) ground turkey**

*Plant-based fat:* **1 tablespoon extra-virgin olive oil**

*SASS:* **¼ teaspoon minced garlic and ½ teaspoon Italian herb seasoning**

Preheat the oven to 350°F.

Cut the tops off the peppers, and remove the seeds and membranes. Set aside. Sauté the onions and garlic in the olive oil until the onions are translucent. Add the carrots, spinach, celery, and herbs, and sauté until tender. Mix in the rice and turkey. Fill the peppers with the turkey mixture, cover with foil, and bake at 350°F for fifteen minutes. Remove the foil, and continue to bake for another five minutes.

## Mediterranean Minted Turkey Salad

*Produce:* **1 cup field greens; ¼ cup each artichoke hearts (canned or jarred in water, drained and rinsed, or vacuum sealed), chopped red bell pepper, and chopped onion; and 4 sun-dried tomatoes, minced**

*Whole grain:* **½ cup cooked bulgur, chilled**

*Lean protein:* **3 ounces roasted, baked, or grilled boneless, skinless turkey breast, diced**

*Plant-based fat:* **2 tablespoons jarred black-olive tapenade**

*SASS:* **3 or 4 fresh mint leaves**

Toss the field greens and mint with the tapenade to coat well, and place in a salad bowl. Top with the bulgur, and then the artichoke hearts, pepper, onion, tomatoes, and turkey.

## Herbed Turkey and Spinach "Spaghetti" Bake

*Produce:* **1 cup cooked spaghetti squash, ¼ cup each baby spinach and sliced mushrooms, and ½ cup all-natural marinara sauce**

*Whole grain:* **½ cup cooked red quinoa**

*Lean protein:* **3 ounces cooked extra-lean (99 percent lean) ground turkey**

*Plant-based fat:* **2 tablespoons sliced almonds**

*SASS:* **1 teaspoon Italian seasoning**

Preheat the oven to 350°F.

Toss the cooked spaghetti squash with the quinoa and Italian seasonings. Fold in spinach, mushrooms, marinara, and turkey. Transfer to a small glass dish, sprinkle with the slivered almonds, and bake at 350°F for fifteen minutes. Remove foil and bake another three to five minutes, or until the almonds look toasted.

## Fiesta Pasta Salad

*Produce:* **1 cup baby spinach leaves and ¼ cup each chopped onion, chopped red and green bell pepper, and grape tomatoes, sliced in half**

*Whole grain:* **½ cup whole-wheat pasta spirals**

*Lean protein:* **3 ounces cooked extra-lean (99 percent lean) ground turkey**

*Plant-based fat:* **10 large black olives, sliced**

*SASS:* **¼ teaspoon minced garlic, 2 tablespoons red wine vinegar, 1 tablespoon chopped cilantro, and dash cracked black pepper**

Toss the pasta with the garlic, vinegar, cilantro, and pepper, and then add the vegetables, turkey, and olives. Serve chilled.

## Turkey Pesto Salad

*Produce:* **1½ cups field greens, ¼ cup each chopped cucumbers and chopped green onion**

*Whole grain:* **½ cup sweet corn, fresh, or frozen and thawed, or kernels sliced from 1 medium ear of fresh roasted corn**

*Lean protein:* **3 ounces roasted, baked, or grilled boneless, skinless turkey breast, diced**

*Plant-based fat:* **1 tablespoon jarred roasted red-pepper pesto**

*SASS:* **1 tablespoon balsamic vinegar and dash cracked black pepper**

Toss the diced turkey with the pesto, and set aside. Combine the field greens with the chopped green onion and cucumber, and place in sealable container together with the vinegar and pepper. Seal, and shake well to coat. Place in a salad bowl, top with the corn and turkey, and serve.

## Turkey Almond Pita

*Produce:* ½ cup baby spinach leaves; 1 medium plum tomato, diced; and ¼ cup each sliced celery and minced cucumber

*Whole grain:* ½ whole-grain pita

*Lean protein:* 3 ounces roasted, baked, or grilled boneless, skinless turkey breast, sliced

*Plant-based fat:* 2 tablespoons almond butter

*SASS:* 2 tablespoons balsamic vinegar and dash cracked black pepper

Toss the vegetables with the vinegar and pepper, and set aside. Spread the inside of the pita with the almond butter. Fill with the turkey and veggies, and serve with any extra on the side.

## Ginger Turkey Stir-Fry

*Produce:* ½ cup each red bell pepper, sliced Into strips; chopped carrots; chopped celery; and chopped red onion

*Whole grain:* ½ cup cooked brown rice

*Lean protein:* 3 ounces cooked extra-lean (99 percent lean) ground turkey

*Plant-based fat:* 2 tablespoons walnuts, chopped

*SASS:* 1 tablespoon 100 percent orange juice, 1 tablespoon rice vinegar, ½ teaspoon freshly grated ginger, and 2 tablespoons chopped scallions

In a small dish, whisk together the orange juice, vinegar, and ginger. Add the scallions. On the stove top over medium heat, using nonstick spray, sauté the vegetables with ginger sauce until the peppers and onions are slightly tender. Add the turkey to heat through. Spread a plate with brown rice, top with the vegetable mixture, and garnish with the chopped walnuts.

## seafood meals

### Tuna-Stuffed Tomatoes

*Produce:* **4 small vine-ripened tomatoes, ½ cup baby spinach, and ⅛ cup each finely chopped green onion and finely chopped celery**

*Whole grain:* **½ cup cooked quinoa, cooled**

*Lean protein:* **3 ounces chunk light tuna canned in water, drained**

*Plant-based fat:* **2 tablespoons walnuts, chopped**

*SASS:* **2 tablespoons balsamic vinegar, 1 tablespoon lemon juice, ¼ teaspoon minced garlic, and dash cracked black pepper**

Slice the tops off the washed tomatoes, scoop out seeds with a melon baller, and set aside. In a large bowl, toss the spinach, green onion, celery, and quinoa with the vinegar, lemon juice, garlic, and pepper. Fold in the tuna and walnuts. Stuff the tomatoes with the quinoa mixture, chill, and serve.

### Salmon Ginger Rice Bowl

*Produce:* **½ cup each sliced red pepper, chopped carrots, and shredded purple cabbage and ¼ cup each chopped celery and chopped onions**

*Whole grain:* **½ cup cooked wild rice**

*Lean protein:* **3 ounces cooked wild salmon**

*Plant-based fat:* **2 tablespoons black sesame seeds**

*SASS:* **1 tablespoon 100 percent orange juice, 1 tablespoon rice vinegar, ½ teaspoon freshly grated ginger, and 2 tablespoons chopped scallions**

In a small dish, whisk together the orange juice, vinegar, and ginger, and then add the scallions. On the stove top over medium heat, using nonstick spray, sauté the vegetables with the ginger sauce until the pepper slices are slightly tender. Fill the bottom of a salad bowl with the rice. Top with the sautéed vegetables and then the salmon, and garnish with the sesame seeds.

### Shrimp Creole

*Produce:* **¼ cup each chopped onion, chopped green pepper, and chopped celery, and 1 cup canned diced tomatoes**

*Whole grain:* **½ cup cooked brown rice**

*Lean protein:* **3 ounces cooked shrimp**

*Plant-based fat:* **1 tablespoon extra-virgin olive oil**

*SASS:* ½ teaspoon minced garlic, ⅛ teaspoon chili powder, 1 teaspoon Italian seasoning, dash cracked black pepper, dash cayenne pepper, and 1 wedge fresh lemon

On the stove top over medium heat, sauté the onions, peppers, and celery in the olive oil until the onions are translucent. Stir in the tomatoes, chili powder, Italian seasoning, and two kinds of pepper. Bring to a quick boil, and simmer about eight to ten minutes. Remove the sauce from heat. Place the rice on a plate, topping with the shrimp and a squeeze of fresh lemon. Top the shrimp with the tomato sauce and serve.

## Citrus Salmon Salad

*Produce:* 1 cup field greens and ½ cup each chopped red onion and chopped green beans
*Whole grain:* ½ cup sweet corn, fresh, or frozen and thawed, or kernels sliced from 1 medium ear of fresh roasted corn
*Lean protein:* 3 ounces cooked wild salmon
*Plant-based fat:* ¼ medium avocado, chopped
*SASS:* 1 tablespoon red wine vinegar, 1 teaspoon Italian herb seasoning mix, and ½ teaspoon grapefruit zest

Toss the field greens with the vinegar and herbs. Transfer to a salad bowl and top with the onions, green beans, corn, and salmon, and garnish with the grapefruit zest.

## Mediterranean Shrimp Pizza

*Produce:* 1 cup baby spinach; ½ cup each chopped red bell pepper and chopped onion; and 4 sun-dried tomatoes, minced
*Whole grain:* ½ whole-grain pita, sliced widthwise, not lengthwise (slice along edge of round)
*Lean protein:* 3 ounces cooked baby shrimp
*Plant-based fat:* 1 tablespoon extra-virgin olive oil
*SASS:* ½ teaspoon minced garlic and ½ teaspoon Italian herb mix

Preheat the oven to 450°F.
Lay the pita, outer side facing up, on a piece of foil and rub with half the olive oil. Sauté the spinach, peppers, and onions with the garlic, herbs, and the remaining olive oil. Top pita with the spinach mixture and then the shrimp, and garnish with the minced sun-dried tomatoes. Bake at 450°F for five to eight minutes.

## Fish Tacos with Cilantro-Jalapeño Guacamole

*Produce:* 1 cup fresh spinach and ½ cup each chopped onions and grape
tomatoes, sliced in half, and ¼ cup low-sodium vegetable broth
*Whole grain:* 2 soft taco-size whole-corn tortillas
*Lean protein:* 3 ounces cooked wild pollack
*Plant-based fat:* ¼ medium avocado, mashed
*SASS:* Dash freshly ground cracked black pepper; 1 teaspoon fresh, chopped
cilantro; 1 small jalapeño, diced, and wedges of fresh lime

Mix the pepper, cilantro, and jalapeño into the avocado to make a guacamole, and
chill. On the stove top over medium heat, sauté the spinach, onions, and tomatoes in
the broth until tender. Warm the tortillas, fill with the fish and sautéed vegetables
(serve extra vegetables on the side), garnish with fresh-squeezed lime juice, and
top with the guacamole.

## Tuna Pecan Pasta

*Produce:* 1 cup chopped green beans; ⅓ cup each chopped onion, chopped
mushrooms, and shredded carrots; and ¼ cup low-sodium vegetable broth
*Whole grain:* ½ cup cooked whole-grain penne
*Lean protein:* 3 ounces canned chunk light tuna, in water, drained
*Plant-based fat:* 2 tablespoons pecans, finely chopped
*SASS:* ½ teaspoon garlic and ½ teaspoon Italian herb mix

Preheat the oven to 400°F.
On the stove top over medium heat, sauté the vegetables in the broth with the
garlic and herbs until the onions are tender. Toss with the tuna and pasta. Transfer
to a small baking pan, sprinkle with the chopped pecans, cover with foil, and bake at
400°F for ten to twelve minutes.

## Lemon Thyme Scallops

*Produce:* 1 cup grape tomatoes, sliced in half, and 1 cup cooked spaghetti
squash
*Whole grain:* ½ cup cooked wild rice
*Lean protein:* 4 ounces raw sea scallops
*Plant-based fat:* 1 tablespoon extra-virgin olive oil
*SASS:* ½ teaspoon minced garlic, 1 teaspoon fresh or ¼ teaspoon dried
thyme, 1 tablespoon fresh lemon juice, and dash crushed red pepper

On the stove top over medium heat, warm half the olive oil. Add the garlic and scallops, and sauté about four minutes on each side. Add the thyme, cook until the scal-

lops are firm and opaque, and then drizzle with lemon juice. In a separate pan, sauté the tomatoes in the remaining olive oil. Toss the spaghetti squash with the rice, and add the sautéed tomatoes. Transfer the squash mixture to a plate, top with the scallops, and dust with the pepper.

## Shrimp Pesto Salad

*Produce:* **1 cup field greens and ½ cup each shredded zucchini and shredded carrots**

*Whole grain:* **½ cup sweet corn, fresh, or frozen and thawed, or kernels sliced from 1 medium ear of fresh roasted corn**

*Lean protein:* **3 ounces cooked shrimp**

*Plant-based fat:* **1 tablespoon jarred basil pesto**

*SASS:* **2 fresh lemon wedges and dash cracked black pepper**

Place the greens, zucchini, and carrots in a sealable bowl. Add the pesto, close the lid, and gently shake to coat thoroughly. Transfer to a salad bowl. Add the corn, top with the shrimp, dust with pepper, squeeze with fresh lemon, and serve.

## Sicilian Sardine Pasta

*Produce:* **2 plum tomatoes, diced, and ½ cup each chopped onions and sliced mushrooms**

*Whole grain:* **½ cup cooked whole-grain penne**

*Lean protein:* **1 3¼-ounce tin sardines in spring water, drained**

*Plant-based fat:* **1 tablespoon extra-virgin olive oil**

*SASS:* **1 teaspoon garlic, 1 tablespoon Italian seasoning, and pinch crushed red pepper**

Chop the sardines and set aside. On the stove top over medium heat, sauté the vegetables and garlic in the olive oil until the onions are tender. Add the Italian seasoning and chopped sardines to heat through. Place the cooked pasta on a plate and cover with the vegetable-and-sardine mixture. Sprinkle with crushed red pepper if desired.

## vegan meals

### Tomato, Basil, and Walnut Salad with Cannellini Beans

*Produce:* 2 medium vine-ripened tomatoes, thinly sliced
*Whole grain:* ½ cup cooked wild rice, chilled
*Lean protein:* ½ cup cannellini beans
*Plant-based fat:* 2 tablespoons walnuts, chopped
*SASS:* 1 tablespoon balsamic vinegar and 3 or 4 fresh basil leaves, chopped

Place the wild rice on a plate. Cover with alternating layers of tomato and cannellini beans. Garnish with the chopped basil, drizzle with the balsamic vinegar, and top with the chopped walnuts.

### Mediterranean Lentils over Couscous

*Produce:* 1 cup fresh spinach, ½ cup each chopped plum or vine-ripened tomatoes and chopped onions
*Whole grain:* ½ cup cooked whole-wheat couscous, warmed
*Lean protein:* ½ cup cooked lentils
*Plant-based fat:* 1 tablespoon extra-virgin olive oil
*SASS:* ½ teaspoon garlic and dash cracked black pepper

On the stove top, warm the olive oil in a pan over medium heat. Add the spinach and onions, stirring until spinach is wilted and onions are translucent. Then add the tomatoes, garlic, and lentils to heat through. Cover a plate with the warmed couscous, top with the lentil mixture, and dust with pepper.

### Chilled Lentil and Wild Rice Salad

*Produce:* 1 cup torn romaine or field greens, ¾ cup diced fresh vine-ripened or plum tomato, and ¼ cup diced white onion
*Whole grain:* ½ cup cooked wild rice, chilled
*Lean protein:* ½ cup cooked lentils
*Plant-based fat:* ¼ medium avocado, diced
*SASS:* 1 tablespoon lemon juice, dash cracked black pepper, 1 tablespoon balsamic vinegar, and 3 or 4 fresh mint leaves, torn

Mix the lemon juice and pepper with the vinegar, and then toss with the greens, tomatoes, onions, and mint. Transfer to a serving bowl, and top with the rice and then the lentils and avocado.

## Edamame Cashew Ginger Stir-Fry

*Produce:* ½ cup each sliced red bell pepper, chopped carrots, and shredded purple cabbage; and ¼ cup each chopped celery and chopped onions

*Whole grain:* ½ cup cooked brown rice

*Lean protein:* ½ cup shelled edamame

*Plant-based fat:* 2 tablespoons cashews, chopped or crushed

*SASS:* 1 tablespoon 100 percent orange juice, 1 tablespoon rice vinegar, ½ teaspoon freshly grated ginger, and 2 tablespoons chopped scallions

In a small dish, whisk together the orange juice, vinegar, and ginger, and then add the scallions. On the stove top over medium heat, using a nonstick spray, sauté the vegetables with the ginger sauce until the peppers are slightly tender. Add the edamame to heat through. Spread a plate with brown rice, top with the vegetable mixture, and garnish with the cashews.

## Black Bean Tacos with Cilantro-Jalapeño Guacamole

*Produce:* 1 cup fresh mushrooms, chopped; ½ cup each fresh spinach and onions, any type, diced; and ¼ cup low-sodium vegetable broth

*Whole grain:* 2 soft taco-size whole-corn tortillas

*Lean protein:* ½ cup canned, rinsed black beans

*Plant-based fat:* ¼ medium avocado, mashed

*SASS:* Dash freshly ground cracked black pepper; 1 teaspoon fresh, chopped cilantro; 1 small jalapeño, diced; and wedges of fresh lime

Mix the pepper, cilantro, and jalapeño into the avocado to make a guacamole, and chill. On the stove top over medium heat, sauté the vegetables in the broth until tender. Warm the tortillas, fill them with the black beans and sautéed vegetables, garnish with freshly squeezed lime juice, and top with the guacamole. Serve any extra vegetables on the side.

## Chickpea and Red Quinoa Lettuce Wraps

*Produce:* **5 large outer romaine leaves and 1 medium vine-ripened or plum tomato, diced**

*Whole grain:* **½ cup cooked red quinoa, chilled**

*Lean protein:* **½ cup chickpeas**

*Plant-based fat:* **10 large black olives, sliced**

*SASS:* **1 tablespoon lemon juice and ½ teaspoon minced garlic**

Toss the quinoa, chickpeas, tomatoes, and olives with the lemon juice and garlic. Fill the romaine leaves with the mixture, and serve.

## Peppery Broad Beans over Vegetable Barley

*Produce:* **1 small red pepper, sliced into strips; 1 cup fresh spinach; and ¼ cup low-sodium vegetable broth**

*Whole grain:* **½ cup cooked barley**

*Lean protein:* **½ cup canned, rinsed broad beans (fava beans)**

*Plant-based fat:* **1 tablespoon jarred basil pesto**

*SASS:* **Crushed red pepper and 1/8 teaspoon ground white pepper**

Toss the broad beans with the pesto, and set aside. On the stove top over medium heat, sauté the peppers in the broth until the peppers are tender. Add the spinach, stirring until wilted. Spread a plate with the barley, and top with the vegetables and broad beans.

## Layered Bean Dip with Cilantro-Jalapeño Guacamole

*Produce:* **5 celery stalks and 1 small red pepper, sliced into thick strips**

*Whole grain:* **½ cup sweet corn, fresh, or frozen and thawed, or kernels sliced from 1 medium ear of fresh roasted corn**

*Lean protein:* **½ cup vegetarian refried beans, warmed**

*Plant-based fat:* **¼ medium avocado, mashed**

*SASS:* **Dash fresh ground cracked black pepper; 1 teaspoon fresh chopped cilantro; 1 small jalapeño, diced; and wedges of fresh lime**

Mix the pepper, cilantro, lime juice from fresh wedges, and jalapeño into the avocado to make a guacamole, and chill. Place the warmed beans in a small bowl. Top the beans with the corn and then the guacamole, and serve as a dip for the red-pepper strips and celery stalks.

---

## slow down to slim down

You've heard it before, but research confirms it: eating more slowly can help you eat less.

A study of more than three thousand men and women published in the *British Medical Journal* concluded that speedy eaters are three times more likely to be overweight than their slower-paced counterparts. A study from the University of Rhode Island found that slow eaters took in about four more ounces of water and 65 fewer calories per day—four times fewer calories per minute than speed-eaters. Fast eaters reported a lower level of satiety, despite eating more food in less time.

Instead of wolfing down your lunch in the five minutes before a meeting, give yourself enough time to eat your meal at a leisurely pace. Try to spend at least twenty minutes eating each meal. Put your fork down or take a sip of water between bites, and focus on really tasting your food. It sounds so obvious, but it's a trick most of us don't use!

---

## Zesty Bean and Summer Slaw Pita

*Produce:* 1 cup shredded cabbage and ½ cup each shredded carrots and chopped red onion

*Whole grain:* ½ whole-grain pita

*Lean protein:* ½ cup canned, rinsed great northern beans

*Plant-based fat:* ¼ medium avocado, mashed

*SASS:* 2 tablespoons rice vinegar, 1 tablespoon 100 percent orange juice, dash cracked black pepper, and ½ teaspoon celery seed

Toss the beans with the avocado, and set aside. Mix the cabbage, carrots, and onions with the vinegar, orange juice, pepper, and celery seed to make a slaw. Fill the pita with the avocado-and-bean mixture and the slaw, and serve, with extra slaw on the side.

## Peppers with Polenta and Pine Nuts

*Produce:* **1 medium green bell pepper, sliced into strips; 1 medium red bell pepper, sliced into strips; and ¼ cup low-sodium vegetable broth**

*Whole grain:* **½ cup (¼ tube) organic polenta**

*Lean protein:* **½ cup lima beans, fresh, or frozen and thawed**

*Plant-based fat:* **2 tablespoons pine nuts**

*SASS:* **1 teaspoon minced garlic and 1 tablespoon fresh or 1 teaspoon dried basil**

On the stove top over medium heat, sauté the peppers in the broth until tender, and set aside. Add the polenta, lima beans, garlic, and basil to a saucepan to heat through. Spread a plate with the seasoned polenta, and top with the sautéed peppers and then the beans. Garnish with pine nuts.

# 5

24 25 26 27 28 29 30 31 32 33

# your daily
# chocolate escape

When my clients come to me for a weight-loss plan, the comment I hear most is: "Just so you know, I can't live without chocolate." Guess what? Neither can I!

I love chocolate so much that I indulge every afternoon. Sometimes it's a truffle I've made myself; other times, it's a square of my favorite organic extra-dark bar. But my personal affection for chocolate isn't the reason I've made a Chocolate Escape your fifth meal of the day. A daily fix of chocolate—dark chocolate, to be specific—is an important part of my plan because of two facts confirmed by research: dark chocolate controls food cravings, and it's good for your health.

Does that sound too good to be true? It's not. Consider what happened in a Danish study when volunteers fasted for twelve hours and then ate three ounces of either dark or milk chocolate with equal calo-

It felt really decadent to eat chocolate. I've always been a perfectionist about diets. If I feel like I have cheated, I go off it. I finally "get" that the chocolate escape doesn't blow the whole diet and ruin the day.

CHRIS, AGE 54

rie levels. Every thirty minutes for the next five hours, the volunteers rated their hunger and fullness levels, their food cravings, and how well they liked the chocolate. Two and a half hours after eating the chocolate, the volunteers were offered pizza and told to eat until they felt satisfied. The upshot? Compared with the milk-chocolate eaters, the dark-chocolate group consumed 15 percent fewer pizza calories and reported that the chocolate made them feel less like eating sweet, salty, or fatty foods.

I've seen this same response among my clients (and myself!). That's why on this plan, dark chocolate is built in as a delicious daily craving crusher. Every day I want you to enjoy 50 to 100 calories' worth of at least 70 percent dark chocolate. In my experience, that's the perfect dose to satisfy and control your cravings and treat your body to chocolate's health benefits.

You can eat individually wrapped squares, many of which are in 50- to 100-calorie portions; buy 200-calorie bars and eat a quarter to a half each day; or make dark chocolate yourself by following the truffle recipes I created especially for this plan. You'll find the recipes starting on page 146. Each recipe takes just five minutes to make and yields a batch of five 70-calorie chocolates. I have created five versions, one using each type of SASS so you can sneak in even more flavor, aroma, and antioxidants.

## the rules for eating chocolate

You can enjoy your Chocolate Escape at any time of the day. There are just two requirements. You must:

- Eat your chocolate without any distractions. This means no TV, no computer, no conversations.

- Let the chocolate melt in your mouth, and savor every morsel. Close your eyes if you want to! Let this be your moment, just for you.

## the history of chocolate

I love to learn about the origins of my favorite foods, and chocolate has a rich history. The ancient Mayans discovered cacao trees in the rainforests and transplanted them on their own lands. Cacao trees produce fruit pods, and the seeds found in these pods are used to make chocolate. Mayans harvested, fermented, and roasted the seeds and then ground them into a paste, which they mixed with water, chili peppers, cornmeal, and other spices to make a spicy chocolate drink. They also used cacao seeds as offerings to their gods and traded them with the Aztecs, who highly valued the cacao drink for its health-enhancing effects. The Aztecs used cacao medicinally for more than one hundred ailments, including fatigue, digestive problems, anemia, fever, gout, and seizures. They considered cacao the "food of the gods" and introduced it to Spain after the Spanish conquest.

The Spanish created their own beverage with cacao, adding sugar, cinnamon, and other spices, and its popularity in Europe grew. Many Europeans believed that a chocolate drink could improve sleep, aid digestion, purify the blood, and act as an aphrodisiac. In London, chocolate houses opened long before coffee shops, but the industrial revolution changed the history of chocolate forever.

Machines allowed chocolate to be mass-produced quickly, and instead of being used as a beverage, cacao was transformed into sweet candy bars, cakes, and ice cream. Unfortunately, the processing added calories and diluted the health benefits, and cacao began to undergo alkalization, a process that is still used today with some chocolates. Alkalization makes cacao less acidic, giving it a milder flavor, but the process significantly reduces the antioxidant content. One study found that natural cacao packed ten times more antioxidants than alkalized, and another found that the antioxidant levels in natural cacao were four times greater than cacao that had been "Dutched," or processed with alkali.

For the best-quality and highest-antioxidant chocolate, look for lightly sweetened, non-"Dutched" cacao. In bars and chips, the only ingredients should ideally be dark chocolate, sugar, and vanilla.

# why chocolate is a feel-good food

Chocolate is one of those foods most people cannot live without. Ninety-one percent of American women crave chocolate, according to a Cornell University study, and there's absolutely no substitute. Chocolate contains unique natural substances, including some that truly create a sense of euphoria. A chemical called phenylethylamine is the very same substance that your brain releases when you fall in love. Another, called anandamide, triggers the same receptors in your brain cells as THC, the psychoactive chemical in marijuana. A third chemical, theobromine, stimulates the heart, relaxes blood vessels, boosts circulation, and has been studied for its possible aphrodisiac effects.

Have you ever found yourself turning to chocolate when you're feeling blue—and then quickly perking up? That's because chocolate appears to boost levels of serotonin and dopamine, brain chemicals involved in regulating your mood. It also has been proposed that women crave chocolate when they're short on magnesium, a mineral that can help alleviate PMS symptoms, including cramps, water retention, fatigue, depression, and irritability.

I like the truffles even better when they sit in the fridge for a few days!
AMY, AGE 28

Not only can chocolate put you in a better frame of mind, but it also may stimulate your mind to operate at a higher level. When Norwegian scientists studied the effects of chocolate, wine, and tea on the cognitive performance of more than two thousand seniors, they found that compared with the seniors who abstained from all three, those who consumed even one—chocolate, wine, or tea—scored significantly higher on challenging brain teasers. The common thread is the antioxidants called flavonoids. What's more, according to Swiss research, chocolate has the power to help correct imbalances in the body related to stress and can significantly reduce levels of stress hormones.

## the buzz about chocolate and caffeine

If you're sensitive to caffeine, rest assured that a daily dose of dark chocolate won't leave you bouncing off the walls. Compared with coffee and tea, chocolate is relatively low in caffeine. One ounce of 70 percent dark chocolate contains up to 40 mg of caffeine, compared with up to 200 mg in eight ounces of brewed coffee and up to 120 mg in strong black tea.

## a daily dose of chocolate can save your life

In addition to making you feel good, several studies show, chocolate offers outstanding benefits to your cardiovascular system. The antioxidants in cocoa powder trigger the walls of your blood vessels to relax, lowering blood pressure and improving circulation. Chocolate's natural substances also help prevent cholesterol from sticking to your artery walls, reducing your risk of heart attack and stroke.

One study found that heart-attack survivors who ate chocolate just twice a week over a two-year period cut their risk of dying from heart disease threefold. Another reported that when women ate dark chocolate for just seven days, their levels of "bad" LDL cholesterol dropped by 6 percent, and their levels of HDL, the "good" kind, rose by 9 percent.

Dark chocolate, in moderation, also may help maintain low levels of inflammation, lowering the risk of clogged arteries. An Italian study published in the *Journal of Nutrition* studied the link between dark chocolate and blood levels of C-reactive protein (CRP), a marker for

# MY STORY

### Cat Chez, 50 | Pounds lost: 10

## While Dieting the Month Before Cinch! I Lost Only 3.5 Pounds Eating Less Food!

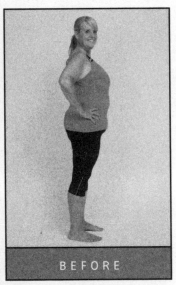

BEFORE

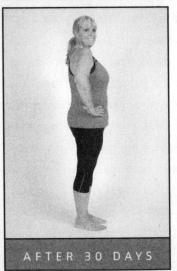

AFTER 30 DAYS

I have been on a lifestyle change for most of 2010, and I thought that I was pretty well educated about nutrition and weight loss prior to starting this plan, but I am a NEW person because of Cinch!

Although I had been dieting for months prior to Cinch!, I was stuck at the same weight for three weeks.

I'm a mom of four kids and a wife and I work, but I've been able to whip up my Cinch! meals fast. At the start of the plan I chose my meals for the next two weeks and stocked up with groceries, and it was super easy. I even bought some special culinary tools as Cinch! brought out the kitchen diva in me I never knew existed! I rearranged a few drawers and added things like new graters, a juicer tool, a garlic masher, and many more measuring cups.

Cynthia introduced me to new concepts that made all the difference and helped me break through my plateau. Before Cinch! I had managed to keep my calorie intake low, but I wasn't always getting the right portions of my foods. For example, I had a lot of difficulty with veggies—I would get bored because I was always reaching for the same ones. This plan opened my world up to enjoying so many more veggies and I love the ability to have them raw. The structure and timing rules also gave me the discipline to NOT pick during the day. Through Cinch! my body has become more regular. I feel like I finally have complete balance!

My Cinch! meals draw a lot of curiosity from friends. I'm a DJ, and usually one of the perks is being able to eat the food at the event, but now I bring my own food. At one of my gigs everyone was inquisitive about my meal. One friend said, "Yummy, all my favorite foods." My husband enjoys the many foods I have been cooking too, so I'm happy I will be able to keep him healthy. I tried out as many of the recipes as I could and they kept surprising me with how amazing they taste! And my daily chocolate escape: I savored it, ate it slowly, let it melt in my mouth. Absolutely delicious!

Bottom line: this plan is AWESOME. I would tell anyone to try it—it really is a Cinch! When you first read some of the meals, you may think you won't enjoy it, but your palate will be surprised. I have not enjoyed food this much ever! And the best part is it's easy.

I am feeling amazing with this plan and feel as though it can take me through my lifetime. I had my oldest daughter over yesterday so she shared in all my meals with me and LOVED THEM. I really believe you have set up the right equation that equals a long and healthy life!

Cinch! has taken me to a new level of good health. When I reached the 150s on the scale I was ecstatic. I haven't seen that number in almost 10 years. I now realize I will reach my goal of 135, which I haven't been in my adult life, and Cinch! has taken away the struggle. Being good at eating right wasn't easy for me, and now it is. I feel like I am just going to continue on the downward spiral—on the scale that is! Woo-hoo!

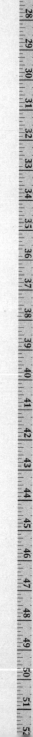

---

## fair trade chocolate

Whenever possible, I buy chocolate that is Fair Trade certified. There are 5 to 6 million cacao farmers worldwide, and 40 to 50 million people depend on cacao for their livelihood, primarily in Africa, Asia, Central America, and South America. Fair Trade certification ensures that the cacao was produced under fair working conditions and in an environmentally sustainable way that preserves the farmland and ensures that farmers are given a fair price, allowing them to invest in their farms and communities and lift themselves out of poverty. Fair Trade–certified cacao products are available at retailers such as Whole Foods Market, Price Chopper, Fred Meyer, Giant, Kroger, and Wegman's. For more information, visit http://transfairusa.org.

---

inflammation. Among the more than forty-eight hundred healthy volunteers, some thirteen hundred had eaten chocolate during the previous year, and more than eight hundred regularly ate dark chocolate. The researchers found that the dark-chocolate eaters had lower CRP levels. Those who ate up to one small daily serving—less than an ounce every three days—had 17 percent lower CRP levels than people who either abstained from chocolate or ate large quantities.

Chocolate may be a remarkably effective way to keep your blood pressure under control. A study published in the *Journal of the American Medical Association* found that among a group of men and women with above-optimal blood pressure, eating just one square of dark chocolate daily for eighteen weeks was enough to reduce the prevalence of high blood pressure in the group from 86 percent to 68 percent.

In addition, chocolate may lower heart-attack and stroke risk by preventing blood clots. In a study published in *Preventative Cardiology*, scientists looked at 139 people who had been disqualified from a larger study on aspirin because they reported eating foods, including dark chocolate, that could have affected the aspirin study's results. As it turned out, the chocolate eaters' blood took longer to clot.

Despite all this research about heart health, you may wonder: isn't chocolate full of unhealthy fat? Not at all. It's true that dark chocolate contains a fair amount of saturated fat; one-quarter cup of dark chocolate chips packs about eight grams of saturated fat. However, the saturated fat in dark chocolate isn't the same as the artery-clogging saturated fat in a hamburger or whole milk. It's a unique variety called stearic acid, much of which gets converted in the body into oleic acid, a heart-healthy monounsaturated fatty acid that lowers "bad" LDL cholesterol and raises protective HDL. Because of this, studies suggest, stearic acid has little effect on levels of "bad" blood cholesterol.

In fact, in my plan, dark chocolate counts as a plant-based fat, which is why—in addition to indulging in your daily Chocolate Escape—you

## the magic of coconut oil

In chapter 2, I discuss the health benefits of coconut oil, including its ability to boost calorie and fat burning, increase HDL cholesterol (the "good" kind), and shrink your waistline. But those aren't the only reasons I include this flavorful oil in some of my truffle recipes.

Like chocolate, coconut oil contains a healthy type of saturated fat, called *lauric acid*. Unlike olive oil and other plant-based oils, coconut oil has a chemical structure that makes it solid at room temperature—yet it dissolves easily, even upon touch. This unique texture is a perfect match for chocolate because the truffles harden quickly and hold their shape, and both chocolate and coconut oil melt on your tongue. Coconut oil also adds a decadent layer of flavor and blends perfectly with both sweet and savory ingredients. I combine it with natural almond butter to give the truffles a bit more stability (so they won't melt in your hand), round out the flavor, and add a dash of protein, minerals, and vitamin E.

can also enjoy dark chocolate at breakfast. My favorite is the Chocolate Pear Ginger Smoothie, found on page 97. If you'd like to experiment with creating your own chocolate meals, see chapter 6 to learn how much to include and what foods to pair it with.

## whip up your own chocolate escape

In just five minutes you can create your own batch of melt-in-your-mouth dark-chocolate truffles. I've incorporated one of the SASS seasonings into each recipe for an extra splash of flavor and antioxidants. Choose any flavor you like, and enjoy one truffle each day, or experiment by substituting the seasonings I've chosen with your own blends. There are so many herbs and spices to choose from; your only limit is your imagination! Wrap the extras in wax paper, and store in a sealable container in your refrigerator or freezer.

### Balsamic Truffles

¼ cup semisweet chocolate chips
½ tablespoon natural almond butter, at room temperature
½ tablespoon extra-virgin coconut oil, at room temperature
1 teaspoon balsamic vinegar

1. Rinse a glass bowl in the sink. Pour out the water, but don't dry the bowl. Place the chocolate chips in the bowl, and microwave for fifteen seconds. Stir, and return for another five to ten seconds if needed.
2. Stir in the almond butter and coconut oil, and then fold in the vinegar. The mixture should form a uniform "batter."
3. Pick up the batter in your hands, and pat it into a round ball.
4. Pinch off five uniform-size pieces, and pat each into a round "truffle."
5. Place on wax paper, and refrigerate for at least fifteen minutes.
6. Wrap the extra truffles in wax paper, place in a sealable container, and store in the refrigerator.

## Citrus Zest Truffles

¼ cup semisweet chocolate chips
½ tablespoon natural almond butter, at room temperature
½ tablespoon extra-virgin coconut oil, at room temperature
½ teaspoon (packed) freshly grated tangerine zest

1. Rinse a glass bowl in the sink. Pour out the water, but don't dry the bowl. Place the chocolate chips in the bowl, and microwave for fifteen seconds. Stir, and return for another five to ten seconds if needed.
2. Stir in the almond butter and coconut oil, and then fold in the tangerine zest. The mixture should form a uniform "batter."
3. Pick up the batter in your hands, and pat it into a round ball.
4. Pinch off five uniform size pieces, and pat each into a round "truffle."
5. Place on wax paper, and refrigerate for at least fifteen minutes.
6. Wrap the extra truffles in wax paper, place in a sealable container, and store in the refrigerator.

## Spicy Chipotle Truffles

¼ cup semisweet chocolate chips
½ tablespoon natural almond butter, at room temperature
½ tablespoon extra-virgin coconut oil, at room temperature
½ teaspoon ground chipotle seasoning

1. Rinse a glass bowl in the sink. Pour out the water, but don't dry the bowl. Place the chocolate chips in the bowl, and microwave for fifteen seconds. Stir, and return for another five to ten seconds if needed.
2. Stir in the almond butter and coconut oil, and then fold in the chipotle seasoning. The mixture should form a uniform "batter."
3. Pick up the batter in your hands, and pat it into a round ball.
4. Pinch off five uniform-size pieces, and pat each into a round "truffle."
5. Place on wax paper, and refrigerate for at least fifteen minutes.
6. Wrap the extra truffles in wax paper, place in a sealable container, and store in the refrigerator.

## Green Tea Truffles

¼ cup semisweet chocolate chips
½ tablespoon natural almond butter, at room temperature
½ tablespoon extra-virgin coconut oil, at room temperature
½ teaspoon loose green-tea leaves (it's okay to tear open a tea bag and use
the leaves; just be sure to measure them)

1. Rinse a glass bowl in the sink. Pour out the water, but don't dry the bowl. Place the chocolate chips in the bowl, and microwave for fifteen seconds. Stir, and return for another five to ten seconds if needed.
2. Stir in the almond butter and coconut oil, and then fold in the tea leaves. The mixture should form a uniform "batter."
3. Pick up the batter in your hands, and pat it into a round ball.
4. Pinch off five uniform-size pieces, and pat each into a round "truffle."
5. Place on wax paper, and refrigerate for at least fifteen minutes.
6. Wrap the extra truffles in wax paper, place in a sealable container, and store in the refrigerator.

## Peppercorn Truffles

¼ cup semisweet chocolate chips
½ tablespoon natural almond butter, at room temperature
½ tablespoon extra-virgin coconut oil, at room temperature
7 twists fresh grated peppercorn

1. Rinse a glass bowl in the sink. Pour out the water, but don't dry the bowl. Place the chocolate chips in the bowl, and microwave for fifteen seconds. Stir, and return for another five to ten seconds if needed.
2. Stir in the almond butter and coconut oil, and then fold in the pepper. The mixture should form a uniform "batter."
3. Pick up the batter in your hands, and pat it into a round ball.
4. Pinch off five uniform-size pieces, and pat each into a round "truffle."
5. Place on wax paper, and refrigerate for at least fifteen minutes.
6. Wrap the extra truffles in wax paper, place in a sealable container, and store in the refrigerator.

# 6

24 25 26 27 28 29 30 31 32 33

# the do-it-yourself
# 5-piece puzzle

**M**any of my clients enjoy making the meals in chapter 4 exactly as described so they don't even have to think about what and how much to eat and how to put it all together. Because I have created one hundred meals for this book, you shouldn't be short on variety, even after you complete your thirty days. However, there may be times when you don't have access to these foods—when you're at a restaurant, for example—or when you simply feel like eating something else. And so I am devoting this chapter to teaching you the very specific structure that I have used for every meal in this book. Once you learn the system, you can understand and visualize how to put meals together when you're away from home, and you can create an endless variety of delicious new meals of your own.

My system is simple. Think of each meal as a "puzzle" constructed from five pieces:

1. Produce
2. A whole grain
3. Lean protein
4. Plant-based fat
5. SASS

The configuration of every meal is identical, except that the produce for breakfast and snacks consists of fruit, and the produce for lunch and dinner is a vegetable.

I have chosen this configuration because I believe it provides the absolute best proportion of carbs, protein, and fat for weight loss, blood-sugar control, and satiety, as well as a broad spectrum of nutrients and antioxidants that you need to look and feel your best. This consistent, fixed meal structure means you'll never have to count calories. It also ensures that every day you'll eat a specific number of servings from each food group. That means you won't end a day without fitting in at least two servings of fruit and four servings of veggies. You also won't miss out on protein, whole grains, or good-for-you fats, because they're built into every breakfast, lunch, dinner, and snack. And each meal is perfectly portioned to give you quick, easy, and sustainable weight loss.

Looking at each meal as a puzzle helps you immediately understand where you may have been off track before following Cinch! For example, many of my clients already were combining whole grains, veggies, and protein at their meals, but their proportions were out of balance, with too few veggies and larger-than-needed amounts of rice or chicken. The perfect proportion of these ingredients gives your body just what it needs to shed extra weight and make it super efficient.

One client's staple meal was a "healthy" vegetarian burrito made with a whole-wheat flour tortilla, brown rice, black beans, shredded cheese, veggies, and avocado. She was right on track with the ingredients but off track with the balance. The tortilla and brown rice together supplied all the whole grains she needed for the entire day, and the black beans and cheese added up to too much protein for one meal—enough to create a surplus that wound up feeding her fat cells. And although she thought she was eating plenty of veggies, when she actually measured, she was getting only three-quarters of a cup in her burrito. Her new Cinch!-style Mexican meal was just as satisfying and what I often refer to as "Goldilocks" size—not too little, not too much, but just right: 2 cups of greens and raw veggies topped with ½ cup corn as the whole grain, ½ cup black beans as the lean protein, and, filling the plant-based-fat slot, guacamole made from one quarter of a medium avocado mashed with lime juice, jalapeños, and cilantro.

In this chapter I lay out the nitty-gritty details of my puzzle, including the list of foods that fall into each food group and how much counts as one serving. I used these exact lists to create the meals in this book. You can do the same to design your own meals or decide what to order when you're at a restaurant. Here's how to do it.

**1. Start with produce.** Choose either something that's in season or something you're craving. When you buy seasonal, locally grown fruits and veggies, they're allowed to achieve their peak ripeness, nutritional value, and flavor; you won't get these benefits from produce that has been picked early and artificially ripened, since it's shipped hundreds or thousands of miles from where it was grown. I love thinking up different ways to use a fruit or veggie while it's available fresh at my farmer's market, and by the time it's out of season, I'm ready to move on and explore the next set of crops. There's just nothing like crisp summer cucumbers, a crunchy fall apple, or fresh spring asparagus. But if you're really craving blueberries in the middle of January, grab a frozen bag and plan the rest of your meal around them.

**2. Add a whole grain.** Run through your list, and decide which grain makes a good fit for your fruit or veggie. This is where texture and temperature come into play. Do you want to combine cooked veggies with

## restaurant meals that solve the puzzle

Most of my clients don't cook every meal at home, so when they dine out, whether it's at a quick-serve or sit-down restaurant, I recommend that they choose establishments that allow them to easily follow the rules of this plan. Here are examples that fit the bill from five major chains.

### CHIPOTLE: MEXICAN

Order: Vegetarian Fajita Burrito Bowl with lettuce and corn salsa—no rice, no cheese, no sour cream

How it fills the puzzle: Produce (fajita veggies, lettuce, and salsa), whole grain (corn), lean protein (black beans), plant-based fat (guacamole, which comes with this dish), SASS (lots! the salsa, beans, and guacamole are all seasoned).

### P. F. CHANG'S: CHINESE

Order: Salmon Steamed with Ginger with brown rice

How it fills the puzzle: Produce (shiitake mushrooms, bok choy, tomatoes, and asparagus), whole grain (brown rice—you'll get more than you need, so stick with a half cup, the size of half a baseball), lean protein (salmon), plant-based fat (oil used in sautéing), SASS (this dish is made with fresh ginger and other seasonings).

hot, fluffy quinoa or pair fresh salad greens with crisp, crunchy whole-grain crackers?

**3. Choose your lean protein.** Think of your protein as more of an accent to a meal than the main event. Scan the list, and think about which protein complements your produce/whole-grain duo. Most proteins are like a pair of black pants—they go with just about anything! For example, top your quinoa and cooked veggies with a half cup of edamame, or garnish your salad with three ounces of cooked shrimp.

**4. Pick your plant-based fat.** Fat lends flavor and texture to the meal

## ROMANO'S MACARONI GRILL: ITALIAN

Order: Grilled Chicken Spiedini with whole-wheat penne

How it fills the puzzle: Produce (roasted vegetables), whole grain (whole-wheat penne—eat just a half cup, the size of half a baseball), lean protein (chicken breast), plant-based fat (extra-virgin olive oil), SASS (this dish is made with fresh lemon zest, rosemary, and other seasonings).

## RUBY TUESDAY: AMERICAN

Order: Smart Eating Creole Catch with steamed broccoli and brown-rice pilaf

How it fills the puzzle: Produce (steamed broccoli), whole grain (brown-rice pilaf—again, the portion is more than you need, so stick with a half cup, the size of half a baseball), lean protein (tilapia), plant-based fat (oil used for broiling), SASS (this dish is made with Creole spices).

## PANERA BREAD: AMERICAN

Order: You Pick Two—Half Classic Café Salad and Black Bean Soup with Whole Grain Baguette, side portion

How it fills the puzzle: Produce (salad is made with baby field greens, romaine, cucumber, red onion, and tomato), whole grain (whole-grain baguette side portion), lean protein (black beans), plant-based fat (oil-based balsamic vinaigrette), SASS (balsamic vinegar in the vinaigrette as well as garlic, lemon juice, and other seasonings in the soup).

---

and generally serves as either the "condiment," like sliced almonds over a salad, or the means to cook or dress veggies—for example, the extra-virgin olive oil used to sauté spinach or dress it as a salad.

**5. The secret weapon: Choose your SASS.** Which of the five seasonings adds the pep or kick that brings it all together? Remember, it's okay to use more than one. I love to make salad dressings with balsamic vinegar, blood-orange juice, garlic, and fresh basil or with lime juice, cilantro, and minced jalapeño.

Using this system, you can modify any restaurant order to make it Cinch! friendly. It's a five-piece mix and match. The goal is to make sure that each piece is there, in the right amounts, with no "extras."

## visualizing your serving sizes

You can't always measure your food or ingredients, so it's helpful to have a visual idea of various serving sizes. I like to use common household objects as a comparison, because they're items you've seen many times, may have around your house right now, and have probably held in your hand. As you're getting used to this plan, I highly recommend gathering some of these objects and placing them in a basket on your kitchen countertop. The more you see and handle them, the easier it will be to estimate their size when you're at a restaurant.

1 cup = a baseball

¼ cup = a golf ball

3 ounces = a deck of cards or a checkbook

1 tablespoon = your thumb, from where it bends to the tip

## take the "my size" quiz: how to customize this plan for your body

When I created this plan, I used my nutrition-science calculators to determine the ideal number of servings per day from various food groups based on the average adult. But as a nutritionist, I know that one plan can't fit everyone's needs. The number of servings of whole grains, protein, and other foods you need is based on several factors, including your age, height, sex, and activity level. So a woman who is five feet, four inches tall, fairly inactive, and thirty-nine years old shouldn't follow the same plan as a five-foot-eight twenty-three-year-old jock who works out five days a week or a five-foot-ten fifty-year-old man.

Creating customized meal plans in a book is a difficult task, but I've designed a way to help you tailor this plan to your body's needs. To find out whether you should increase or decrease the size of your meals, take this brief "My Size" quiz.

> 24 25 26 27 28 29 30
>
> The lack of hunger amazes me. I think I am waking up to exactly how much I used to eat, and it is rather shocking!
>
> RENEE, AGE 45

Questions: *Give yourself one point for every yes response, zero for each no:*

1. For women, are you over five-foot-four? For men, are you over five-foot-nine-and-a-half?

2. Do you have more than fifty pounds to lose?

3. Does your job require that you stand or move for more than four hours per day?

4. Do you fit in cardio-type exercise more than thirty minutes per day at least five days per week?

5. Do you engage in strength training at least twice per week?

6. Are you under forty years of age?

7. Would you describe your metabolism as fast (you have a difficult time gaining weight, and you lose weight easily)?

8. Do you work irregular hours (not on a set schedule) or shifts other than nine to five?

9. Do you regularly get eight hours of sleep per night?

10. Do you watch less than one hour of television per day?

11. Would you describe your stress level as low?

12. Do you feel that you are highly aware of your body's physical sensations of hunger and fullness?

Score: _____

If you scored:

Zero to four points—A low score indicates that you may need to slightly scale back this plan. After the 5-Day, 5-Food Fast Forward, modify the twenty-five-day Cinch! core plan by omitting the whole grain from your snack. Choose snacks that can easily be modified in this way. For example, leave the oats out of the Pineapple Almond Peppercorn Parfait and the Strawberry Vanilla Hazelnut "Ice Cream," and omit the corn from the California Sunshine Salad.

Five to seven points—This plan should be right on track for your needs.

Eight to twelve points—A high score indicates that you may need to bulk up this plan to better fuel your body. Double the whole-grain portion of your breakfast and lunch. For example, use a half cup dry oats instead of a quarter at breakfast, and a whole pita rather than a half at lunch.

Whether or not you modify this plan, be sure to monitor your hunger and fullness signals. If you feel more than a moderate level of hunger, or if you start feeling physical hunger signals more than an hour before your scheduled meal, use a trial-and-error approach to tweak your plan. Even slight changes in the portion sizes of one or two pieces of the puzzle can be enough to help you achieve that "Goldilocks" feeling. For more about moderate versus intense hunger, revisit pages 17 and 20 in chapter 1.

## zero-prep cinch! core meal kits

Life happens! I realize that some days are incredibly hectic, and you may not be able to plan and prepare real meals each day. For occasions when I'm traveling, on the go, or feeling a major time crunch coming on, I keep on hand a handful of packaged, prep-free meals as my emergency backups.

The first is Lärabar fruit and nut bars. They're made simply, from all-natural fruit and nuts, with no sweeteners, flavors, or other additives, and they're absolutely delicious. I don't know how they do it, but one of my favorite flavors, Cashew Cookie, contains only cashews and dates (that's it!) but really does taste like a cookie. You can use any flavor Lära-bar bar you'd like to fill the fruit and plant-based-fat pieces of the puzzle at breakfast or snack time. They're available nationwide in grocery and drugs stores, at amazon.com, or at larabar.com.

When fresh veggies and lean protein just aren't a possibility, I rely on a brand called Just Tomatoes, Etc. They sell packages and minitubs of dried vegetables, both organic and conventional, with zero additives (hence the "Just" in their name). I always keep Organic Just Crunchy Carrot Bits for veggies and Organic Just Soy Nuts for lean protein on hand. You can buy them at retail stores such as Whole Foods, at amazon.com, or at justtomatoes.com.

My favorite on-the-go whole grain is a brand of crackers called Doctor Kracker. They make snack-size bags (one-ounce pouches) of delicious whole-grain crackers that are available at amazon.com or drkracker.com. (Seedlander is my favorite.)

For plant-based fat, my favorite product is Justin's. They make tear-open pouches that hold exactly 2 tablespoons of organic or natural nut butters in nine different flavors, including Classic Almond, Classic Peanut Butter, and Chocolate Hazelnut Butter. One even has the SASS built in: Cinnamon Peanut Butter. You can stock up at retail stores and at amazon.com or justinsnutbutter.com.

Finally, for other portable SASS options, I rely on an amazing company called Tsp Spices. They sell a wide range of seasonings in portable, 1 teaspoon tear-open packets. I always keep organic-ginger pouches in my purse to sprinkle into hot or cold water or tea. Tsp Spices sells everything from single seasonings, including basil and chili pepper, to spice blends like Mull This Over,

> 24 25 26 27 28 29 30
>
> I am amazed at how poorly I was planning my meals. I was living on processed food. This is much better, much more satisfying and much more invigorating. I have more energy throughout the day, and my clothes feel looser.
>
> LAURENE, AGE 36

which contains orange zest, cinnamon, cardamom, lemon zest, allspice, and cloves. You can purchase them at amazon.com or tspspices.com.

In a pinch, you can partner up these healthy, packaged products to make a complete meal, and they're all available at amazon.com. Think of them as your Cinch! first-aid kit.

## breakfast and snack

1 Lärabar bar, any flavor (fills fruit and plant-based-fat puzzle pieces)

¼ cup Just Tomatoes, Etc. organic soy nuts (fills lean-protein puzzle piece)

1 Doctor Kracker snack bag (fills whole-grain puzzle piece)

1 Tsp Spices packet (fills SASS puzzle piece)

## lunch and dinner

¼ cup Just Tomatoes, Etc. dried veggies and ¼ cup Just Tomatoes, Etc. dried soy nuts (fills veggie and lean-protein puzzle pieces)

1 Doctor Kracker snack bag (fills whole-grain puzzle piece)

1 packet Justin's nut butter (fills plant-based-fat puzzle piece)

1 Tsp Spices packet (fills SASS puzzle piece)

# putting the puzzle together
## fruit

I love fruit, but many of my clients shun the sweeter side of produce out of fear that the carbs, sugar, or glycemic index make it "fattening." Others think it's okay to skimp because they double up on veggies. In truth, fruit is an essential element of a healthy diet. Studies show that fruit eaters have lower body mass indexes, even more so than veggie eaters, and fruits are chock-full of nutrition. Yes, they contain sugar, but it's natural sugar bundled with dozens of essential nutrients, including fiber, vitamins, minerals, and antioxidants.

That's one of the reasons veggies alone don't cut it. Banning fruit drastically narrows the spectrum of nutrients your body is exposed to, including many tied to the pigments responsible for fruits' vibrant hues. One Colorado State study found that the women who ate a wider array (eighteen botanical families instead of five) of the exact same amount of produce for two weeks showed significantly less oxidation, a marker for premature aging and disease. (For a refresher on oxidation, see page 105.)

As for the glycemic index, which is essentially a measure of how a food impacts blood-sugar and insulin levels, that number for most fruits is actually low to moderate. Fifty-five or less is considered low; grapes score a forty-three, strawberries a forty, pears and oranges a thirty-three. And the glycemic index plummets when fruit is combined with protein and healthy fats, which it always is in my plan, because both nutrients slow the digestion and absorption of a meal.

One of the U.S. government's main health goals has been to increase to 75 percent the proportion of Americans who eat at least two servings of fruit daily. Right now only 33 percent meet this goal. Achieving a daily double can help you slash the risk of nearly every chronic disease, including heart disease, stroke, certain cancers, and type 2 diabetes. Because one serving of fruit is included at every breakfast and snack, this plan assures that you'll always get two servings—every single day.

### One Fruit Serving Equals
- 1 cup fresh or frozen
- 1 medium piece, about the size of a baseball
- ½ cup canned, in natural juice (no added sugar)
- ¼ cup dried, unsweetened, or sweetened with 100 percent fruit juice

NOTE: What's in season may vary based on where you live, but I've included the general seasons for each selection. To find out where your local farmer's market and pick-your-own farms are, check out www.localharvest.org.

Apples (fall, winter)
Avocados (year-round)
Berries (summer)
Dates (winter)
Grapefruit (winter)
Kiwi (summer)
Limes (spring, summer)
Melons (spring, summer)
Oranges (winter)
Peaches (summer)
Pineapple (fall)
Pomegranate (fall, winter)
Tangerines (winter)

Apricots (spring, summer)
Bananas (year-round)
Cherries (summer)
Figs (summer)
Grapes (summer, fall)
Lemons (year-round)
Mangoes (spring)
Nectarines (summer)
Papayas (year-round)
Pears (fall, winter)
Plums (summer)
Strawberries (spring, summer)
Watermelon (summer)

## variety: a secret disease-fighting strategy

Many of my clients who strive to eat more fruits and veggies wind up eating the same few varieties over and over, but eating a wide variety is just as important as getting enough.

Fact ————————————————————————————————

Just one extra serving of fruit per day can slash your risk of cancer by 6 percent.

Instead of buying a bag of apples, buy three different-colored apples (red, yellow, and green) as well as a few fruits you've never tried before.

A wider variety of produce, even at the same total quantity, offers a big advantage, because it provides a broader spectrum of antioxidants that go to work in your body. I have woven a wide variety of fruits and veggies into this plan, but I encourage you to mix it up even more. Aim for produce from at least three different color families a day, and try meals made with varieties you don't typically eat.

## why i love dried fruit

Dried fruit definitely doesn't deserve the bad rap it's been saddled with. Many people tell me they pass it up because it's "fattening" and loaded with sugar, but that's not true, at least not if you choose the right kind. Drying fresh fruit can cause a loss of vitamin C, but fresh fruit also loses vitamin C every day after it's been harvested, and in general, drying is a good way to preserve nutrients and antioxidants.

If you took a cup of grapes and removed most of the water, you'd get about a quarter cup of raisins. Nothing has been added, and all that has been taken away is moisture. That means a quarter cup dried is the nutritional equivalent of one cup fresh. In fact, if you added the moisture back, the fruit would return to its original shape.

The main purpose of drying is to remove the moisture from fruit so bacteria, yeast, and mold can't grow to spoil the fruit or make you sick. Drying also slows down the action of the enzymes naturally found in fruit that cause it to ripen, so the process extends the fruit's shelf

I really feel that this plan is a dream! I am feeling great, really thinking about what I eat and when, and learning how to prepare meals in a new way. I love cooking and trying new things!

JESSICA, AGE 32

# MY STORY

## Sally Andrea, 32 | Pounds lost: 9

## I Became a Healthy Role Model for My Son!

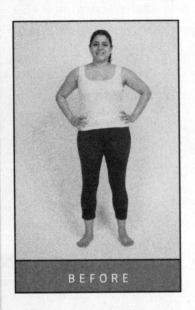

BEFORE

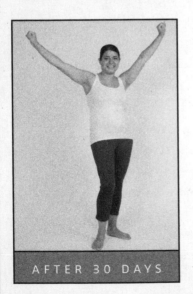

AFTER 30 DAYS

I have been battling with my weight loss for almost three years now since I was pregnant and have never been able to lose more than three pounds. Instead, dieting had caused me to gain ten-plus pounds! Before Cinch! I had tried so many diets, and although they were all legitimately healthy, they were never easy to follow, and I lost focus.

Cinch! is by far the easiest, most appetizing, and most rewarding concept I have ever found. It's the easiest because it's simple. It's the most appetizing because it's not extreme—not just all protein or no fruit. It has a little bit of everything, so if I'm craving chicken and pasta, I can eat it, or if I want rice and beans, I can eat it. And it's the most rewarding because I feel the mental, physical, and emotional difference.

My head is more clear because I don't overstuff myself during lunch. My body is lighter because I'm making healthier choices. And my emotions are more controlled because my sugar levels don't spike and drop. And, oh, the chocolate escape … I don't think I need to explain how great that piece of this plan is. :)

I feel spectacular in more ways than one. I wake up looking forward to having my first meal of the day. My appetite holds strong until lunchtime (which used to be very rare), and as a result, I am able to restrain myself from eating poorly. I look forward to my little snack, which breaks up the day and holds my appetite until dinner, and my light dinner gives me a restful and easy night's sleep. I definitely feel my blood sugar leveling out, and I'm losing pounds and inches.

The puzzle concept soon became second nature. I know what to piece together and how foods go best together, but most important, I now understand what combinations are ideal (e.g., don't eat corn and brown rice in the same meal as that is too many whole grains). I like the fact that I have restrictions that won't allow me to veer off. For example, eating up to a certain amount of points a day is just too vague to me. This plan is more regimented, but you still have a certain amount of flexibility.

Because I'm so busy between work, home, and family, I sometimes get lazy about being creative with my meals. But even when my food isn't as exciting as Cynthia's recipes I don't *have* to use her recipes and it still works… that's the beauty of it! And I can eat out and still feel good. Whenever I ate at Chipotle in the past, I needed a nap. Now I'm able to eat at a place I love but I know how to make better choices.

I would tell anyone considering this plan that this is the easiest lifestyle change you can make, whether you're a stay-at-home mom or an on-the-go power woman. The reason I know is because when I'm home, I am easily able to implement it, and when I'm at work, it's even easier. When I'm busy traveling, the pieces of the puzzle are all around (a bag of nuts at the airport, an apple . . . ), and when I'm busy with my son, I'm still able to follow it.

This is a new way of eating, and I am loving it!

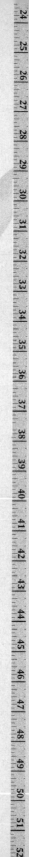

life. Some manufacturers add sugar or corn syrup and preservatives like sulfur dioxide, but these additives aren't needed.

My rule of thumb is to buy dried fruit only with no added ingredients, but there are a few exceptions. Because some berries, such as cranberries, can be bitter, a small amount of 100 percent fruit juice (usually apple juice or apple-juice concentrate) is sometimes added. But many brands add sugar, so watch out! In some cases, dried fruits are lightly misted with sunflower oil or another liquid vegetable oil to prevent them from clumping together. That's okay. Just check the ingredient list. All you should see is the fruit itself, or at the very most, the fruit, a pure fruit juice or juice concentrate for sweetening, and possibly a natural liquid oil.

These days you'll find both traditional dried fruit (technically called "dehydrated"), which tends to retain some moisture and have a chewy texture, and freeze-dried options. The main difference is that before it's dried, freeze-dried fruit is frozen, just as the name implies. After freezing, the fruit is put into a chamber that uses a vacuum to gradually remove the water content while it thaws. The end product has all the flavor and nutrition of fresh fruit, but with a crispy, dry texture.

Both dried and freeze-dried fruits have a long shelf life, but in general, freeze-dried versions keep much longer. Dried fruits tend to lose their taste and flavor after about a year, whereas freeze-dried berries can be stored for several years if they're sealed in an airtight container and kept away from moisture.

## vegetables

Vegetables are generally defined by what they are not rather than what they are. Technically, a vegetable is a nutritional and culinary term for any part of a plant consumed by humans that's not classified as a fruit, nut, herb, spice, or grain. There are countless health benefits tied to eating your veggies, including a reduced risk of heart disease, type 2 diabetes, cancer, kidney stones, bone loss, and obesity. Most vegetables

Fact ——————————————————————————————————————————

A recent study found that cooking carrots whole and chopping them afterward preserves more flavor as well as an antioxidant called falcarinol, a natural cancer fighter. Cooking carrots breaks down its cells, which makes falcarinol more absorbable. One study found that overall levels of antioxidants in carrots jump by 34 percent after cooking.

——————————————————————————————————————————————

are naturally low in sodium and calories, and none have cholesterol. (Cholesterol is a substance made by the liver of animals, so it's found only in animal-derived foods.) The U.S. government's goal has been to increase to 50 percent the proportion of Americans who eat at least three servings of vegetables daily. Right now, only about 27 percent meet this goal. In my plan, I included two servings of veggies at each lunch and dinner, so you'll rack up four every single day. You'll "one-up" the targeted goal!

One Vegetable Serving Equals
- 1 cup fresh or frozen
- ½ cup of "veggies from the shelf," such as all-natural salsa or tomato sauce or canned, diced tomatoes
- ¼ cup of dried veggies such as sun-dried tomatoes (also see section titled "Zero-Prep Cinch! Core Meal Kits" on page 156)

## the most important vegetables you're not eating

A recent study found that a natural chemical in the cruciferous vegetables—broccoli, cauliflower, Brussels sprouts, cabbage, and kale—protects the blood-vessel bends and branches, areas that tend to be the most prone to cholesterol plaque buildup and inflammation. Previous studies have found that those same veggies contain natural detoxers that can deactivate carcinogens and stop the growth of existing cancer cells.

# artichokes: my favorite leafy green

Artichokes are one of my personal favorite veggies, and in my opinion they're one of the most beautiful veggies on earth. But I've observed many people tentatively pick one up, look at it, and put it back, opting for canned hearts instead, because they're just not sure how to select or cook one.

Trust me: artichokes aren't as tricky as they look! There are several varieties of artichokes, but the most common is the globe artichoke, which is a member of the thistle family and originated in the Mediterranean. Aside from being delicious, artichokes are incredibly good for you. One whole artichoke provides just 25 to 50 calories, depending on its size, along with up to one-fourth of all the fiber you need for the day. Plus, artichokes provide calcium, potassium, folate, vitamin C, and antioxidants.

Look for an artichoke that's slightly tender, with no brown tips. The leaves should be tight, not "blooming," and if you run your thumb over the top of the bud, the leaves should not separate. Next, give it a little squeeze: if it makes a slight squeaking noise, it's fresh. After you buy the right one, if you aren't going to prepare it right away, sprinkle it with water and wrap it in a towel or bag to help maintain its moisture.

Okay, now time to cook it! Here's an easy six-step process for properly cooking a fresh artichoke.

1. Rinse the artichoke well.
2. Cut off the stem and the top one-third of the artichoke.
3. Peel off the smallest outer leaves.
4. Place the artichoke facedown in a glass dish with 2 tablespoons water in the bottom, and cover with wax paper.
5. Cook for seven minutes on high in the microwave.
6. Leave the paper cover on, and let stand for five minutes.

To eat, pull off outer petals, one at a time. Tightly grip the nonfleshy end of the petal. Place it in your mouth and pull through your teeth to remove the soft pulpy portion of the petal. Discard remaining petal. The artichoke tastes fantastic drizzled with balsamic vinegar.

Artichokes (spring)                    Asparagus (spring)
Beets (year-round)                     Bok choy (fall, winter)
Broccoli (fall, winter)                Brussels sprouts (fall, winter)
Cabbage (year-round)                   Carrots (year-round)
Cauliflower (fall, winter)             Celery (year-round)
Cucumbers (summer)                     Eggplant (summer)
Endive (fall, winter)                  Fennel (spring)
Green beans (summer)                   Kohlrabi (fall)
Leeks (winter)                         Lettuce (year-round)
Mushrooms (fall, winter)               Okra (summer)
Onions (year-round)                    Parsnips (fall, winter)
Peppers (year-round)                   Pumpkin (fall)
Radishes (summer)                      Seaweed (year-round)
Snow peas (spring)                     Spaghetti squash (fall, winter)
Spinach (spring)                       Sugar snap peas (spring)
Summer squash (summer)                 Swiss chard (spring)
Tomatoes (summer)                      Turnips (fall, winter)
Watercress (spring)                    Winter squash (fall, winter)
Yellow wax beans (spring)              Zucchini (summer)

## whole grains

Whole grains are a key source of vitamins, minerals, fiber, and disease-fighting antioxidants, and the magic number in this plan is four, as in four servings per day.

There are many types of grains, but the words *whole grain* have a very specific meaning. Grains that are "whole" contain the entire grain kernel, which has three distinct parts: the bran (the outer skin of the kernel), the germ (the inner part of the kernel that will sprout into a new plant), and the endosperm (the germ's food supply and largest portion of the kernel).

Refined grains have been processed, which removes both the bran and germ. Processing gives grains a finer texture and improves their shelf life, but it also removes dietary fiber, iron, and many vitamins. For example, when brown rice is processed into white, up to 90 percent of the nutrients are lost. The average intake of whole grains in the United States is less than one serving per day, and fewer than 10 percent of Americans consume three servings per day. My plan includes one serving at every meal, so you'll finish each day with four.

### One Serving of Grain Equals
- 1 standard-loaf-size slice of whole-grain bread
- ½ whole-grain English muffin or pita
- ½ cup cooked whole grain such as wild rice or whole-wheat pasta
- 2 soft taco-size whole-corn tortillas
- ½ whole-grain flour tortilla
- 1 serving hot or cold whole-grain cereal or crackers (see package for serving size)
- 3 cups popped popcorn

*Single Whole Grains*
Barley
Brown rice
Buckwheat
Bulgur (cracked wheat)
Corn
Oats
Quinoa
Wild rice
Whole-wheat couscous

There are several other whole grains I haven't used in my recipes, simply because the selections on the list above tend to be my personal go-to staples. But you can experiment with many on your own, including the following:

Amaranth
Farro
Kamut
Millet
Rye
Sorghum
Spelt
Teff
Triticale

To learn more about them and how to use these grains, visit www .wholegrainscouncil.org.

*Packaged Options*
Whole-corn tortillas
Whole-grain bread
Whole-grain cereal
Whole-grain crackers
Whole-grain English muffins
Whole-grain or whole-wheat pasta
Whole-grain pita
Polenta
Popcorn

Fact ——————————————————————————————
One study found that people who start every morning with whole grains are 28 percent less likely to develop heart failure, and men with the highest whole-grain intakes were 19 percent less likely to develop high blood pressure compared with those who ate the least.

### the trick to buying whole grains

If you're not accustomed to eating whole grains, it's important to become an avid label reader to avoid being fooled. Foods labeled with the words *multigrain, stone-ground, 100 percent wheat, cracked wheat, seven-grain,* or *bran* may not be whole-grain products. Also, color is not an indication of a whole grain. Bread can be brown because of molasses or other added ingredients. Reading the ingredient list is really the only way to see whether a product is made entirely from whole grains. In a nutshell, millet, amaranth, and oats are always whole grain, but if you don't see the word *whole* in front of *wheat, corn, barley,* or *rice,* these grains have been refined.

**Fact** ———————————————————————————————

The average intake of whole grains in the United States is less than one serving a day. Fewer than 10 percent of Americans eat the minimum recommended three daily servings.

### cool your carbs to burn more calories

Fat-burning carbs? Yes indeed! Carb-rich foods including beans, potatoes, corn, barley, brown rice, and whole-grain pasta are some of the best sources of resistant starch (RS), a filling, fiberlike substance that your body doesn't digest. One study found that replacing just 5.4 percent of total carbohydrate intake with RS resulted in a 20 to 30 percent increase in fat burning after a meal.

Resistant starch forms when starchy foods are cooked and then cooled. Because it's not absorbed, RS travels to the large intestine, where it gets fermented by bacteria. This creates fatty acids that may block the body's ability to burn carbohydrates, causing you to burn fat instead. Animal studies have found that RS also prompts the body to pump out more satiety-inducing hormones. When you choose a meal made with one of these fat-fighting superstars, let it cool a bit before digging in.

### get things moving with fiber

About 80 percent of adults struggle with constipation at some point, and brief periods of irregularity are normal. But when things aren't moving in the right direction, the scale creeps up, and we wind up with cramps and a poochy tummy.

Get things going by upping your intake of soluble fiber. This sticky fiber soaks up water, forming a gel-like substance that stimulates the muscles of your digestive system to contract and push waste through faster. The best sources are oats, beans, barley, and fruit, especially citrus, berries, pears, and apples, all of which are found in the meals and snacks in chapter 4.

## lean protein

Protein is one of the main building blocks in your body. It's part of every cell, including muscles, organs, skin, and hair, and is even a component of nearly every bodily fluid. Protein is essential for growth and development during childhood, adolescence, and pregnancy, but even when we're done growing, we use the protein from food to continuously maintain and heal our bodies.

If too little protein "shows up for work," your body will fall into disrepair, and you'll begin to feel and see the effects, such as a weaker immune system, dry skin, dull hair, and shrinking muscles. Protein also helps to stabilize blood sugar and keep you fuller longer, and protein-rich foods are excellent sources of important minerals, including iron and zinc.

But too much protein, more than your body needs for its maintenance and repair work, can strain your kidneys (which have to excrete the by-products of excess protein) and increase the risk of gout, an agonizing form of arthritis that often strikes the base of the big toe. And the "leftover" calories from surplus protein either cause weight gain or prevent weight loss. To help you consistently achieve the best balance, I have included one serving of protein at every meal. The list of protein options includes vegetarian and animal-based options, but if you're an omnivore (you eat everything), I encourage you to choose at least five plant-based meals per week. This will up your antioxidant intake and enhance your weight-loss results.

**One Serving of Lean Protein Equals (choose organic whenever possible)**

- ½ cup cooked beans or lentils
- 1 cup organic skim milk or milk substitute (e.g., organic soy milk)
- 6 ounces plain nonfat yogurt or yogurt substitute (e.g., soy yogurt)
- ⅓ of a 14-ounce package of extra-firm tofu
- ¼ cup egg whites, 1 large whole egg, or whites from 3 large eggs
- ½ cup nonfat cottage cheese
- ¼ cup nonfat ricotta cheese
- 1 slice reduced-fat cheese
- 1 reduced-fat string cheese
- 1 ounce (¼ cup) reduced-fat shredded or crumbled cheese
- 3 ounces skinless poultry or fresh or frozen seafood
- 3 ounces extra-lean 99 percent ground turkey

*Plant-Based Protein*

Beans and lentils. Any variety, such as azuki, black, black-eyed peas, chickpeas (garbanzo beans), edamame (whole soybeans), fava, great northern, kidney, lima, lupin, mung, navy, pinto, and red; also split peas and brown, green, and red lentils

Coconut milk*

Coconut-milk yogurt*

---

*Coconut milk and coconut-milk yogurt are much lower in protein than soy or hemp milk, but I included them for people who avoid or cannot eat soy and hemp. If you choose them, please be sure to eat plenty of bean- and lentil-based recipes to ensure a higher daily protein intake.

Hemp milk
Organic soy milk
Organic soy yogurt
Organic tofu

*Animal-Based Protein*
Organic eggs
Nonfat organic milk
Nonfat organic cottage cheese
Nonfat organic ricotta cheese
Nonfat organic plain yogurt
Organic crumbled cheeses, such as blue, feta, and gorgonzola,
     reduced fat whenever possible
Pre-portioned cheeses, such as mini Babybel and organic string
     cheese, reduced fat whenever possible
Shredded cheeses, such as organic Asiago, mozzarella, and Parmesan,
     reduced fat whenever possible
Sliced cheese such as organic cheddar, fontina, Gouda, Havarti, Jack,
     Swiss, and Muenster, reduced fat whenever possible
Chicken, boneless skinless breast, 99 percent lean ground
Turkey, boneless skinless breast, 99 percent lean ground
Seafood, including cod, halibut, mackerel, pollack, salmon, sardines,
     scallops, shrimp, and tuna

## plant-based fat

It may seem counterintuitive, but fat is one of the most important nutrients in your diet. Fat is a structural part of every cell membrane in your
body, which means you can't heal a cell or construct a new one without
this key building block. Fats also are a component of skin and hair, and
certain types of fats are essential for controlling blood clotting, keeping
your brain healthy, and fighting inflammation in your body. Without fat,

## slash your cholesterol in one simple step

Oatmeal is found in the pantries of 80 percent of all American households—a good thing, because eating just one bowl of oatmeal a day can lower cholesterol by 8 percent to 23 percent, and each 1 percent drop in serum cholesterol translates to a 2 percent decrease in the risk of heart disease. A lot of people ask me about the difference between quick-cooking oats and steel-cut oats. Both types are whole oats, so there's no need to worry that quick-cooking oats are refined. The only difference is their shape. Steel-cut oats are whole-oat kernels that have been chopped into two or three pieces. Quick-cooking oats have been steamed and rolled to flatten them so they cook instantly when hot water is added.

you wouldn't be able to absorb certain antioxidants and the fat-soluble vitamins—A, D, E, and K—which "hitch a ride" with fat to get transported from your digestive system into your blood.

According to the Institute of Medicine and the National Institutes of Health, up to 35 percent of the calories you eat per day can come from fat. In this plan, I aim for 30 to 35 percent, with an emphasis on plant-based fat. That's because your body reacts differently to different types of fats even at the same calorie level.

Saturated fats, from animal-based foods like whole-milk cheeses and fatty meats, tend to override your body's satiety mechanism, the "I'm full" signals, but plant-based fats help to regulate your appetite and keep your weight under control. They also go to work in your body to lower your "bad" LDL cholesterol, increase your "good" HDL cholesterol, and keep your arteries soft and flexible, reducing the risk of heart attack and stroke.

To help achieve the best balance, I have included one serving of plant-based fat at every meal, from one of five categories: (1) nuts and seeds; (2) olives; (3) avocado; (4) oil; and (5) dark chocolate.

### One Serving of Plant-Based Fat Equals
- 1 tablespoon oil or pesto
- 2 tablespoons nuts (whole or whole and then chopped or crushed), seeds, all-natural nut butters
- 2 tablespoons olive tapenade
- 10 whole green or black olives
- ¼ medium Hass avocado
- ¼ cup semisweet- or dark-chocolate chips

*Nuts and Seeds*
Almonds
Brazil nuts
Cashews
Hazelnuts
Peanuts
Pecans
Pine nuts
Pumpkin seeds
Sesame seeds
Sunflower seeds
Tahini
Walnuts
Butters made from any nut
    or seed listed

*Olives*
Black and green whole olives
Black- and green-olive
    tapenade

*Avocado*
Sliced, chopped, or mashed

*Oils*
Almond
Avocado
Canola
Cashew
Coconut
Flaxseed
Hazelnut
High-oleic safflower
High-oleic sunflower
Macadamia nut
Olive
Peanut
Pecan
Pesto, any variety
Pine nut
Pistachio

Pumpkin seed
Sesame
Walnut

*Dark Chocolate*
Semisweet- or dark-chocolate
chips

### the trans-fat transition

In the 1980s, consumer watchdog groups began nutrition-education campaigns to warn people about the risks of saturated fat. Heart disease had been the number one killer, and the link between the two was becoming clear. Consumers responded, and in turn, food manufacturers began removing saturated fat from food. But they had to replace it with something. And that something was man-made trans fat, otherwise known as partially hydrogenated oil.

The hydrogenation process was developed way back in the 1890s, to turn liquid oil into solid margarine. By 1911, shortening had been invented, but most baked goods were still made with animal fats, including butter and lard. When consumers began demanding the removal of saturated fat, trans fat stepped in. The switch was perfect for food manufacturers, because they could make their customers happy and create products with a longer shelf life. A pie crust made with lard will turn rancid quickly, but one made with shortening could last for months.

> I used to feel overly full or hungry after meals—I was starving or stuffed. But I haven't felt either since beginning Cinch!
>
> TESS, AGE 30

Other foods packed with trans fat include margarine, frozen dinners, fried foods, and packaged foods made with shortening or partially hydrogenated oil, such as some brands of crackers, chips, cookies, and muffins.

Unlike other fats that you can safely include in your diet, trans fats clearly are harmful. Numerous studies have documented the relationship between trans fat and heart disease, which is still the number one killer of

## my favorite protein

If I were stranded on an island and could eat only one food for the rest of my life, I'd pick beans. They are chock-full of protein, fiber, and minerals, and they're hearty and satisfying without making you feel weighted down. Plus, they're versatile: you can eat them hot or cold, whole or mashed, and in savory or sweet recipes. Beans are one of the least expensive foods you can buy, and they're one of the healthiest.

A recent study that followed men and women for nineteen years found that those who ate beans four times per week had a 21 percent lower risk of heart disease than once-a-week eaters. The high fiber content of beans may play a role: one cup (two servings) packs about 50 percent of all the fiber you need for the day!

Regular bean eaters have a lower risk of obesity and smaller waistlines, and some studies score beans higher on the antioxidant charts than blueberries. Dried, frozen, fresh, and canned beans are all good options. If you're worried about sodium, pick up low-sodium canned beans with no added salt. Also, rinsing beans in a colander under the sink can wash away about 40 percent of the sodium.

Americans. Trans fat also has been linked to infertility, cancer, type 2 diabetes, liver problems, and obesity. In a recent study, researchers followed more than eighteen thousand married women with no infertility history for eight years while continuing to assess their diets and their attempts to get pregnant. The scientists found that the women's total fat and cholesterol intakes were not linked to infertility, but infertility risk jumped by a whopping 73 percent with each 2 percent increase in trans fat.

Weight-control studies in animals have found that when the exact same number of extra fat calories are added to the diet, animals gain four times more weight with trans fat than with unsaturated fat. And

## solid versus liquid fat

For years, I have advised my clients about a secret, handy way to distinguish good fats from bad fats: think about which are solid at room temperature. Saturated fats are mostly found in animal-based foods, such as meats and whole-milk dairy products. If you've ever made soup, chili, or stew and let it sit on the stove or countertop, you've probably seen the solid fat that rises to the surface or congeals along the edges. Bacon grease also hardens at room temperature, and if whole milk weren't homogenized (blended together), you'd see that the milk fat would separate and rise to the top. In fact, about 50 percent of an eight-ounce glass (one cup) of farm-fresh whole milk is pure fat, the type used to make cream and butter. Fats that are rigid at room temperature have a chemical structure we refer to as *saturated*. That means the arrangement of the fat molecule allows it to bond with many hydrogen atoms, which makes it more stable and solid.

Most saturated fats are bad for us because they remain pretty solid in our arteries. I ask my clients to imagine pouring extra-virgin olive oil through a straw: it goes right through; whereas bacon grease or butter would clog it up.

But recently scientists have learned that not all saturated fats affect the body in the same way. There are actually some types of saturated fat, including those in coconut and cacao (chocolate), that actually protect the heart. Ninety-two percent of the fat in coconut oil is saturated fat, but studies have show that coconut oil protects "good" HDL cholesterol, boosts calorie and fat burning, and decreases waist sizes. And as I mention in chapter 5, a relatively large percentage of the saturated fat in cacao gets converted to a heart-healthy monounsaturated fatty acid that lowers LDL and raises HDL. And because coconut and cacao are plants, they also contain antioxidants. That's why I've included both as options for the plant-based-fat puzzle piece.

for women with heart disease, eating too many trans fats may increase their risk of dying suddenly from cardiac arrest, according to a Harvard study of eighty-seven thousand women followed for twenty-six weeks. The women who ate the most trans fats—2.5 percent of their daily calories—were three times more likely to die of cardiac arrest than those who ate the least—less than 1 percent of their daily calories. On this plan it's easy to achieve less than 1 percent, since you minimize processed foods.

Based on the evidence, the latest version of the *Dietary Guidelines for Americans* states that the optimum goal for trans-fat intake is as close to zero as possible. Fortunately, food manufacturers must now reveal the amount of trans-fat grams per serving on the Nutrition Facts label. For this reason, and because of increased consumer awareness, more and more manufacturers and fast-food restaurants have removed trans fat from foods. Trans fats are banned in New York City, and other cities across the nation are considering following suit.

But assessing your intake of trans fats is tricky. Technically, a product can claim to provide zero grams of trans fat if it contains less than 0.5 grams per serving. That means that if it actually has 0.4 grams and you eat ten servings, you take in 4 grams, not zero grams, of trans fat. Checking the ingredient list is critical. If the words *partially hydrogenated* appear, bingo!—there's some hidden trans fat in the product.

## worse than trans fat?

Many companies are eliminating trans fats from foods, but they may be replacing them with something that may wind up being worse for your health: interesterified oil, also known as fully hydrogenated oil.

A lot of packaged products, like cookies and pie crusts, require a solid fat to hold the ingredients together. If you've ever made either one with liquid oil, you know what happens: the cookies and pie crusts spread out and don't hold their shape properly, and over time the oil separates out. If crackers were made with liquid oil, they'd probably end up looking like a slew of crumbs sitting on top of a pile of oil.

Fact ──────────────────────────────────────────────
A recent study published in the journal *Cell Metabolism* found that animal-based saturated fats trigger your immune system to pump out toxic molecules that spur inflammation—a known trigger of premature aging and disease.
────────────────────────────────────────────────

So manufacturers found a way to create man-made solid fat that can be called "trans-free." That's because technically, a product can also be labeled trans-free if it's made with fully hydrogenated instead of partially hydrogenated oil. From a chemistry-textbook definition, fully hydrogenated oils are trans-free. But they're not risk free. A Brandeis University study found that eating products made with interesterified oil caused the study subjects' "good" HDL cholesterol to drop and triggered a significant rise in blood sugar, about 20 percent, in just four weeks.

That's a real double whammy health-wise. Having a high level of HDL reduces heart-disease risk because HDL is the "good" cholesterol that transports "bad" LDL cholesterol away from arteries. And having high blood sugar thickens the blood, stresses the heart, strains the kidneys, and interferes with the delivery of oxygen and nutrients within the body, especially to the extremities.

Remember the old saying that there's no such thing as a "free" lunch? I think that definitely applies here. In other words, you just can't have shelf-stable processed foods that are problem free. That's why the best way to avoid *both* partially and fully hydrogenated oils is to eat as many unprocessed or minimally processed foods as possible and always, always read the ingredient list. Be extra careful to check oils for the "H word"— *hydrogenated*—whether partial or full, and the new term: *interesterified.*

## why you won't find margarine or corn oil on the list

Saturated fats and trans fats aren't the only fats I've limited in this plan; I've also restricted some polyunsaturated fatty acids, or PUFAs. Two of the major sources in the typical American diet are margarine and corn oil.

A high intake of PUFA may increase the risk of a painful inflammatory bowel disease (IBD), according to research from the University of East Anglia in the United Kingdom. In a study that included more than two hundred thousand Europeans, those with the highest PUFA intake were more than twice as likely to develop IBD as those who consumed the least. Researchers say excess amounts of PUFA are absorbed into the lining of the colon, where they can promote inflammation, a precursor to disease. The study, which followed people for up to eleven years, showed that those with the greatest PUFA intake were two and a half times more likely to develop IBD than people who consumed the least. There's currently no proven dietary treatment for IBD, but these findings show that limiting PUFAs may be a potent safeguard.

## SASS

As I explain in detail in chapter 3, the seasonings, herbs, and spices in the SASS group contain powerful anti-aging, disease-fighting compounds and also help with calorie control by boosting the flavor and aroma of your foods. Within each of the five categories of these core seasonings, you'll find a wide variety of options—far more than I could even use in the recipes I included in this book. I urge you to experiment with your own combinations. Remember, it's okay—in fact, it's even better—to use more than one in a single meal!

24 25 26 27 28 29 30

I was always getting mad at myself before for overeating, but now I know there was nothing wrong with me. I wasn't getting the proper nutrition, and my brain was telling me I was still hungry because my body wanted the right nutrients. Ah ha!

LAURENE, AGE 36

*Vinegar*
Apple cider
Balsamic
Champagne
Cider
Fruit infused (such as black
    currant, cherry, fig, peach,
    pear, plum, pomegranate,
    nectarine, raspberry, and
    strawberry)
Malt
Red wine
Rice
White

*Citrus Juice and Zest*
Citron (Indian citrus fruit)
Clementine
Grapefruit
Key lime
Kumquat
Lemon
Lime
Mandarin orange
Orange, any variety (navel,
    Valencia, sunburst, honey,
    blood, etc.)
Pomelo (a cross between a
    grapefruit and a navel
    orange)
Tangelo (hybrid of a tangerine
    and either a pomelo or a
    grapefruit)
Tangerine

Ugli fruit (cross between a
    grapefruit and a tangerine)
Yuzu (Japanese citrus)

*Hot Peppers*
Anaheim
Cayenne
Cherry
Chili
Chipotle
Habanero
Jalapeño
Mirasol
Pasilla
Pequin
Pimiento
Poblano (referred to as *ancho*
    when dried)
Scotch bonnet
Serrano
Tabasco
Thai
Tien tsin

*Tea*
Black
Green
Oolong
White

*Herbs and Spices*
Allspice
Anise
Basil

| | |
|---|---|
| Bay leaf | Nutmeg |
| Caraway | Oregano |
| Cardamom | Paprika |
| Celery seed | Parsley |
| Chive | Peppercorn |
| Cilantro | Peppermint |
| Cinnamon | Poppy seed |
| Clove | Rosemary |
| Coriander | Saffron |
| Cumin | Sage |
| Dill | Savory |
| Garlic | Spearmint |
| Ginger | Tarragon |
| Lavender | Thyme |
| Lemongrass | Turmeric |
| Marjoram | Vanilla |
| Mint | |

## learning to use herbs and spices

If you didn't grow up with a fabulous cook who taught you how to make time-honored family recipes using a myriad of herbs and spices, your seasoning repertoire may be a bit limited. Mine was, for years. Even though I have some formal culinary training, I'm not a chef, and knowing which herb or spice to use in what quantity and combination did not come naturally. But as with every skill in life, practice is the key. Each time you build a new meal, think of it as a culinary adventure! Here are a few tips that may help:

- Before adding an herb or spice, smell it. If the aroma seems to blend with the other foods in your meal, try it.
- Start with a small amount, and taste as you go along to judge whether you need to add more.

- For short cooking times, less than fifteen minutes, add seasonings at the beginning.
- For longer cooking times, add your seasonings during the last twenty to thirty minutes.
- When using dried herbs, crush them in the palm of your hand (or between your fingers) before adding to the food to release more flavor quickly. The usual proportion for dried to fresh is to use one teaspoon of dried herbs for every one tablespoon of fresh.
- Limit the use of strongly flavored herbs within a single meal. These include basil, dill, marjoram, mint, rosemary, sage, tarragon, and thyme.
- To crush a small amount of herbs or spices, use a mortar and pestle, which allows you to control the coarseness. For large amounts, use a spice mill or small coffee grinder.

To learn about individual varieties of herbs and spices and how to use them, check out the information and resources at the McCormick Science Institute's website at www.mccormickscienceinstitute.com.

## juicy news about citrus

The Latin word *citrus*—which was borrowed from ancient Greek *kedros*, "cedar, juniper"—refers to trees with fragrant foliage or wood that have no relation to cedar. When I lived in Florida, I had orange and pink grapefruit trees in my backyard, and when they were in blossom, the aroma was intoxicating. Maybe that's why research shows that the scent of grapefruit makes women appear about six years younger to men!

# 5-piece puzzle cheat sheet

Buying organic is recommended but not mandatory. See page 205 for tips on ways to save on organic options.

| PUZZLE PIECE | ONE SERVING EQUALS | NOTES |
|---|---|---|
| Produce | **Fruit:** <br> 1 cup fresh or frozen <br> 1 medium piece, about the size of a baseball <br> ½ cup canned in natural juice (no added sugar) <br> ¼ cup dried, unsweetened, or sweetened with 100% fruit juice <br> **Veggies:** <br> 1 cup fresh or frozen <br> ½ cup "veggies from the shelf," such as all-natural salsa, tomato sauce, or canned, diced tomatoes <br> ¼ cup dried veggies | Fruit at breakfast and snack; veggies at lunch and dinner <br><br> Go for locally grown, in-season produce and choose organic when possible, especially: <br> Celery <br> Peaches and nectarines <br> Strawberries <br> Apples <br> Blueberries <br> Bell peppers <br> Spinach and kale <br> Cherries <br> Imported grapes |
| Whole grain | Must be 100% whole grain: <br> 1 standard-loaf-size slice of bread <br> ½ English muffin or pita <br> ½ cup cooked grain such as wild rice or whole-wheat pasta <br> 2 soft taco-size corn tortillas <br> ½ whole-grain flour tortilla <br> 1 serving (according to package) hot or cold cereal or crackers <br> 3 cups popped popcorn | Millet, amaranth, and oats are always whole grain, but if you don't see the word *whole* in front of *wheat*, *corn*, *barley*, or *rice*, these grains have been refined |

| | | |
|---|---|---|
| Lean protein | **PLANT-BASED:**<br>½ cup beans or lentils<br>⅕ of a 14-ounce package of extra-firm organic tofu<br>1 cup milk substitute (e.g., organic soy milk)<br>6 ounces nondairy yogurt<br>**ANIMAL:**<br>1 cup nonfat organic milk<br>6 ounces plain nonfat organic yogurt<br>¼ cup organic egg whites, 1 whole organic egg, or 3 organic egg whites<br>½ cup nonfat organic cottage cheese<br>¼ cup nonfat organic ricotta cheese<br>1 slice reduced-fat organic cheese<br>1 reduced-fat organic string cheese<br>1 ounce (¼ cup) reduced-fat shredded or crumbled organic cheese<br>3 ounces poultry or seafood | Use organic nonfat milk and yogurt and reduced-fat cheese when possible<br><br>If you're an omnivore, aim for 5 vegetarian or vegan meals per week<br><br>If you're vegetarian, aim for 5 vegan meals per week<br><br>Look for 99% lean ground poultry and skinless poultry |
| Plant-based fat | 1 tablespoon oil or pesto<br>2 tablespoons nuts, seeds, all-natural nut butters<br>2 tablespoons olive tapenade<br>10 whole green or black olives<br>¼ medium avocado<br>¼ cup dark or semisweet chocolate chips | Measure nuts, then chop |

| SASS | No specific serving sizes<br><br>SASS includes:<br>Vinegar<br>Citrus juice and zest<br>Hot peppers<br>Tea (brewed or dry leaves)<br>Herbs and spices | Use vinegar with 15 calories per tablespoon or less; limit to 6 tablespoons per day<br><br>Use a maximum of ¼ cup 100% citrus juice per day as a seasoning<br><br>Limit to 3 whole hot peppers per day<br><br>No limit on fresh or dried herbs and spices<br><br>Use at least 1 of the 5 SASS seasonings at each meal |
|---|---|---|
| Visual references for serving sizes | 1 cup = a baseball<br>¼ cup = a golf ball<br>3 ounces = a deck of cards or checkbook<br>1 tablespoon = your thumb, from where it bends to the tip | |

Emergency Backup Kit Meals:

Breakfast and Snack

1 Lärabar, any flavor (fills fruit and plant-based-fat puzzle pieces)

1 Doctor Kracker snack bag (fills whole-grain puzzle piece)

¼ cup Just Tomatoes, Etc. organic dried soy nuts (fills lean-protein puzzle piece)

1 Tsp Spices packet (fills SASS puzzle piece)

Lunch and Dinner

¼ cup Just Tomatoes, Etc. dried veggies and ¼ cup Just Tomatoes, Etc. organic dried soy nuts (fills veggie and lean-protein puzzle pieces)

1 Doctor Kracker snack bag (fills whole-grain puzzle piece)

1 packet Justin's nut butter (fills plant-based-fat puzzle piece)

1 Tsp Spices packet (fills SASS puzzle piece)

# 7

24 25 26 27 28 29 30 31 32 33

# losing is a cinch!

My husband is really good at computers and technical stuff. Anytime my e-mail stops working, I can't get a video to play online, or I need to update my website, he's there to help. Every once in a while, I'll ask him to explain how something works, and he's happy to do it because he's a self-professed geek who loves tech talk. But as much as I want to understand it, I usually wind up saying, "Never mind," because the answer is just too complicated! The same thing happens in reverse when I try to explain why I don't think he should drink a protein shake right before a workout or why oil-and-vinegar dressing is a better choice than ranch. In situations like this, he'll usually say, "Okay, just tell me what to eat."

As a health professional with extra training in counseling and a former college instructor, I really want my clients to understand every nuance of why I recommend what I do and how it works. But I know that sometimes that's just TMI—too much information. In chapters 4 and 6, I tell you what, how much, and when to eat. Here, you can take your time reading about the logic behind the Cinch! plan, including the research I've used and wisdom I've accumulated in my nearly twenty years of nutritional counseling practice. I address several "why" questions—for example, why I believe calorie counting is outdated, why the timing of your meals affects your weight, and why eating organic and vegetarian can help you shed pounds.

## *why:* not all calories are created equal

Calories are important to weight control, but I've chosen not to make them the focus of this plan. Realistically, nobody wants to go around adding up every single calorie, and sometimes you just don't have that information. Fresh veggies from your local farmer's market don't come with a Nutrition Facts label, so for this plan, I did something a little different that my clients really love. I built the calories into the blueprint by using specific portions of fruits or veggies, whole grains, lean protein, and plant based fat. Because the structure of each meal is fixed and the portion sizes are specific and uniform, your calorie intake will automatically fall into place, right where it should be. And most important, you'll get the most from your calories in the right balance, packed with the right nutrients.

That's important because, despite what you may have heard, not all calories are created equal. If you've ever had a blueberry muffin for breakfast and felt hungry again an hour later, you know exactly what I'm talking about. A typical-size muffin (four ounces) packs 400 to 500 calories. Sitting at your desk working burns about 100 calo-

I bring my afternoon snack to work because I know by the time I get home I am just so super hungry. This is helping me not want to eat the second I get home from work.
JESSICA, AGE 32

ries per hour, so technically, that muffin should fuel you for four to five hours. But it doesn't.

That's because your body handles different types of calories in different ways. Refined grains, which lack fiber and nutrients, and refined sugar both get digested and absorbed quickly. They empty out of your stomach faster and get broken down in your digestive tract and absorbed into your bloodstream quickly. As a result, a big surge of sugar rushes into your blood all at once. This spike triggers your pancreas to secrete insulin, a hormone that gets your blood sugar back into balance by essentially clearing the excess sugar out of the blood and bringing it to your body's cells. That means that within a short period of time, your cells are presented with a large load of fuel. Unless they can use it all at that moment, which is unlikely unless you're out hiking or engaged in an activity that burns several hundred calories an hour, your body has no choice but to shift what it doesn't need to your fat cells.

Your body's active cells (muscles, organs, etc.) need a steady stream of fuel throughout your waking hours to perform their various jobs. If you give them enough calories for several hours' worth of work all at once, there's no "holding area" for the fuel to hang out in. In other words, once it clears the blood and reaches the cell, if it's not needed right then and there, it gets shuffled off to storage—that is, fat land.

This process explains why some people who don't really overeat wind up overweight. A good chunk of a 400-calorie blueberry muffin can end up getting stored as fat within a fairly short period of time, whereas a 400-calorie meal made from whole grains, fresh fruit, lean protein, and good-for-you fat is much more likely to get completely burned off. Fiber, lean protein, and healthy fat all delay stomach emptying, so right away you stay fuller longer and postpone digestion. Fiber, protein, and fat also slow down the absorption of carbohydrates from your GI tract into your blood, so instead of experiencing a big sugar rush, you get a slower, lower rise in blood sugar. That in turn triggers a more controlled release of insulin and a steady delivery of fuel to your cells. This is exactly the kind of pattern your body loves. It gets an even, time-released delivery of fuel as it needs energy throughout your day.

**Bottom-Line Logic:** Balanced meals delivered at the right times match your body's natural rhythm. If you've been out of balance, you'll feel and see a difference within a few days of starting this plan.

## why: calorie counting is outdated

In the past few years, scientists have learned more and more about how our bodies react to identical calorie levels of different foods. One recent study found that saturated fats, like those found in butter, whole milk, and fatty meats, override the body's natural satiety mechanism, whereas unsaturated fats, from plant sources such as olive oil, avocado, and nuts, actually enhance satiety, even when the calorie levels don't differ. Another study, published in *Clinical Nutrition,* found that even at the exact same calorie level, meals made with unsaturated fat from walnuts and olive oil caused a 20 to 30 percent rise in postmeal calorie burning compared with meals made with saturated fat from whole-milk dairy products. And in chapter 3, I mention the University of Florida research showing that people with higher antioxidant intakes from more plant-based foods weigh less and have less body fat even though they eat the same number of calories as people who consume fewer antioxidants.

**Bottom-Line Logic:** Although I don't believe in ignoring calories altogether, the research and my clinical instincts tell me that the quality of every calorie is even more important than the total quantity.

## *why:* meal timing matters

I have briefly explained how meal timing is important for regulating your metabolism. You can probably tell that I'm a fan of analogies, and here's one I always use to illustrate the importance of timing: Imagine you're taking a car trip from New York City to Orlando, Florida. You'd probably make sure you had a full tank before you hit the road, and when your tank started to run low, you'd find a place to fill up for the miles ahead. Cars and bodies have a lot in common in that, ideally, you provide them with energy *proactively.* After all, if you needed a tank of gas to travel five hundred miles, it would be impossible to drive that distance on an empty tank and fill it up when you get there.

That's the biggest difference between your automobile and your body. If your car runs out of gas, it will putter out and stay that way until you reload, but your body can't do that. It's "on" twenty-four hours a day, and because you constantly need fuel to support your heart, lungs, and other vital functions, your body is programmed to adapt to being underfueled. The effects of "running on empty" are actually worse than the effects of eating something unhealthy, like a doughnut. That's because not eating forces your body to make something out of nothing; in other words, when no fuel is available, your body has to adapt. And it does two things: First, it switches into conservation mode and burns fewer calories, which means your energy level stays low and your brain and body don't perform as well as they should. Second, your body dips into your fuel reserves, which include your body's own muscle mass. Over time this loss of muscle can lead to weight gain, because the less muscle you have, the fewer calories you burn. Losing precious muscle also increases your injury risk, because your muscles become worn down and weaker.

Recent research supports the notion that poorly timed meals impact weight—even without an increase in total calories. A study from Northwestern University, published in the journal *Obesity,* looked at two groups of mice over a six-week period. Both groups were fed a high-calorie diet to induce weight gain, but they ate at different times. One group ate at times when they would normally be asleep, and those mice put on twice as much weight, despite engaging in the same amount of physical activity and eating the same amount of food as the other mice.

Scientists have called this study groundbreaking, but throughout my years as a nutritionist I have always believed that it's not just total daily calories consumed that matters but also the relationship between the body's energy demands at the time of the meal and the amount of energy the meal provides. I've had many, many clients who really don't overeat calorie-wise, but they eat 60 percent of their calories between 4:00 P.M. and 10:00 P.M., hours during which they're fairly inactive. I've also seen many people lose weight simply by eating the same number of calories per day but breaking up their total intake into more even chunks that are spaced three to five hours apart.

I always tell my clients that when your body receives calories, there are only three potential fates: (1) the calories get burned, but only if the energy demand is high enough to burn them; (2) the calories get used for repair/maintenance, tasks like healing muscle, replenishing glycogen, and so on, but only if there are repair jobs that need those raw materials; or (3) the calories are sent to fat storage because the fuel and repair needs have been met.

I have been teaching this concept for nearly twenty years, based on what I've learned and what I've seen in my practice. I've heard doctors and even some dietitians say that it doesn't matter when you eat, that it's only your total calories that count. But to me, that simply doesn't make sense, and at least four other studies published within the past five years support the idea that meal timing impacts weight control.

**Bottom-Line Logic:** Breaking up your intake into smaller, evenly timed meals stokes up your body's fat-burning furnace, improves satiety, decreases the chances of rebound overeating at later meals, and results in better control of both blood-sugar and insulin levels and cholesterol.

# MY STORY

### Maleika Cole, 24  |  Pounds lost: 11

## Allover Inches Lost: 10.25.
## I Feel Like I Have My Life Back

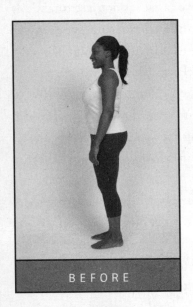

BEFORE

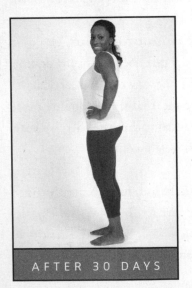

AFTER 30 DAYS

Cinch! came at the perfect time in my life. I work full-time but I'm also an aspiring singer, so I need to look good *and* have energy. For years I have been the quintessential yo-yo dieter, either in "diet mode" or "free-for-all mode," and both are bad places. I've tried bars, shakes, cleanses, packaged meal plans, you name it.

The most weight I ever lost in a week was on a low-carb diet, but I was tired all the time and felt sluggish. I was also bored and my cravings were out of control.

I was tired of being overweight and feeling like a failure, and just plain tired of being tired. I needed a plan that allowed me to have more energy, put really good things in my body, and keep my cravings in check, and that's what Cinch! gave me.

At first I mourned the loss of my best friend food, but I pushed past it and it was one of the best decisions I've ever made. This is the first time in years that I haven't eaten late-night junk food or had terrible cravings or drank alcohol. After just a few days I started to feel like my body was working really well and I was putting in exactly what it needed to function. I also lost my craving for sweets. This plan is so different from every other plan I've followed because it doesn't feel restrictive and it's very clean. And it's so simple—no points or counting.

With other approaches it was easy to miss a protein or a fat. I'd think I was doing well but now I realize that I was depriving my body of essential nutrients. I've never had all of the pieces of the puzzle together until now.

I also learned that eating is a multisensory experience. The dishes Cynthia created are not only easy to prepare and taste great, they are BEAUTIFUL! When something looks pretty, with colors and different textures on the plate, you almost forget about stuffing your face. The food becomes part of an overall experience instead of the main event. And it is so great that you can prepare these meals ahead of time.

Reducing salt makes me feel powerful! Getting rid of the salt shaker has awakened my senses and allowed me to experience *more* flavor from herbs and spices. And I feel like I'm not tempted to overeat when my salt is in check.

With Cinch! it's so easy to piece meals together. I really like the idea of the puzzle. I like that my meal has multiple elements—I don't feel like I'm getting cheated! And now that I'm not always planning my next meal or thinking about food, I'm a happier and more productive person!

What's also very special about Cinch! is that it tackles not just the food, but also the emotional aspects of eating. This is the first time I am approaching food with honesty. With other plans I would always sneak things, but with Cinch! I don't have to—I feel satisfied and food has become nourishment. Before, food was always on my mind. I would go out with people JUST for the food. Now, I am sitting enjoying my friends. WOWSAHS!!!!!

I'm really happy with my thirty-day results, and I'm fully committed to making this my way of life, which means I know I'll lose more. Before this plan, I was headed with full force toward obesity. Cinch! has empowered me to make my health a priority.

If you're just getting started my advice is to follow the plan 100 percent. Don't make up your own rules. Trust me. I tend to be a rule breaker, but I'm so happy I didn't this time. Cinch! really works. I feel like I have my life back.

## *why:* nutrient balance is key

The analogy I like best to explain nutrition and weight loss is to think of your body as a construction project, like a house. In order to build a house, an architect needs to draw up a blueprint that sketches out the exact amount of raw materials needed (wood, concrete, plumbing, etc.), along with specific calculations and instructions for how to put it all together. Without a blueprint, you could easily wind up with, well, one big mess.

Nutrition is similar. Every day, your body needs a specific amount of carbohydrate, protein, fat, vitamins, minerals, antioxidants, and water to keep your structure—your body—in perfect working order. In a nutshell, every cell in your body, from a lung or muscle cell to a red blood cell, performs a job, and those cells need water, fuel, and nutrients to carry out their jobs properly. In addition, cells get stressed, they're constantly subjected to wear and tear, and eventually they die off. Getting the right types of nutrients in the right balance, in the right amounts, and at the right times will allow your body to perform at its best, heal properly, and continually renew itself.

When your diet is out of balance, you're giving it either too little or too much. Taking in too few nutrients can zap your energy, because you're not providing enough fuel to meet your body's needs. A nutrient shortage also can prevent your body's cells from performing their jobs optimally, slow the healing of stressed or damaged cells, or stop your body from replacing cells that have died off. When you fall short on nutrients, you'll eventually feel or see the effects. Some of the common symptoms include sluggishness, bloating, constipation, mood swings, dull or dry hair and skin, and a weak immune system. I want to ensure that all the nutrients you need show up for work in your body every single day, in the right amounts, to keep you in perfect physical working order. In all of my years as a nutritionist, I've never had a client who wasn't lacking something that the body needed. Filling in the gaps, even small ones, can make a major difference in how much weight you lose and how quickly.

## poor meal timing triggers rebound eating

A recent study found that among people with a forty-hour workweek, an eight-hour stretch between meals resulted in a 40 percent jump in calorie intake. The longer people waited, the more they overate at the next meal and the more they chose lower-quality, less nutritious food.

On the flip side, when too many nutrients show up for work, you run into a different set of problems. Taking in too many calories from any food (even veggies!) gives you an overall surplus, and any excess fuel your body doesn't need either gets socked away in your fat cells, causing you to gain weight, or supports the excess fat you already have, keeping it on your body.

That last part can be a little confusing, but here's how it works: Once you've gained excess fat, you need to keep feeding the fat in order to maintain it. On average, it takes about 10 calories to support every extra pound of body weight for an inactive person. Think of it as a math formula. If it takes 1,500 calories to keep you at 150 pounds and you begin eating 1,600, you'll eventually get to 160 pounds, but you'll have to keep eating 1,600 calories a day to maintain that 10-pound weight gain. This formula explains why some people hit a weight-gain plateau, meaning they had been gaining and gaining and suddenly their weight stabilizes. That happens when the number of calories they're eating on a daily basis is only enough to keep them at the plateau weight, but not enough to cause any additional weight gain.

Most Americans actually have an under/over problem—they fall short on some important nutrients and eat excess amounts of others.

That's why it is possible to be vitamin deficient and overweight at the same time. It takes a balance of nutrients for you to reach your ideal weight and optimal body function.

**Bottom-Line Logic:** When I sat down to formulate this plan, I knew it had to supply enough nutrients to meet your body's needs in the right balance. It also had to provide only enough calories to support your ideal weight. Remember, in order to keep the excess body fat you've gained, you have to eat enough calories to support it. The "fixed" structure of this plan (the five-piece puzzle) doesn't allow that, so by following the plan, you'll shrink your size to get to and stay at your weight goal. The structure also ensures that by the end of the day you get a specific number of servings from each food group, including two fruits and four veggies.

## another reason not to nix carbs

Cutting out high-carb grains and fruits altogether may lead to weight loss, but it also slashes your intake of the important nutrients they pack, including fiber and antioxidants. The average American gets only about half of his or her recommended fiber per day; fiber not only helps with digestion and lowering cholesterol but is also a major weight-control tool.

Fiber fills you up but supplies no calories to your body because you can't digest or absorb it. One study of Brazilian dieters found that over a six-month period, each additional gram of fiber eaten daily resulted in an extra quarter-pound weight loss. Other research has shown that for every gram of fiber you eat, you eliminate roughly 7 calories. That means that eating twenty-five grams of fiber each day essentially cancels out nearly 200 calories from your diet; that alone could be enough to allow you to shed twenty pounds over the course of a year.

Feeling super this morning, actually nice and hungry. I forgot what a great feeling that is.

CHRIS, AGE 54

---

## there's a new "you" every day

Every cell in your body has an average life span. Stomach-lining cells live about 2 days, the cells that line your intestines 3 days, skin cells about 28 days, red blood cells 120 days, liver cells 200 days, and brain cells up to 50 years. Your body is always building new cells to take the place of the ones that have died off, and those cells are made directly from the nutrients in your diet. In essence, your body is like a very complex construction site.

---

Whole grains, including brown rice, oats, and barley, also are chockfull of fiber and antiaging, disease-fighting antioxidants. Corn, for instance, has almost twice the antioxidant activity of apples, while oats rival broccoli and spinach in antioxidant activity. Bottom line: it's all about balance. Rather than cutting out carbs altogether, this plan simply cuts down on them and emphasizes the most healthful carbs so you get the most nutrition bang for your bite.

## *why:* more vegetarian meals mean more weight loss

Elsewhere in the book I cover some of the ways that eating more plant-based foods can help you lose weight. In chapter 3, for example, I mention a study that links more antioxidants from plant-based foods to better satiety and lower body weights, even without a reduction in calories.

Overweight and obesity rates in the general population have been skyrocketing. According to the Centers for Disease Control and Prevention, 67 percent of American adults age twenty and over are overweight or obese. Currently 26.4 percent of men and 24.8 percent of women are obese. Yet the prevalence of obesity among vegetarians and vegans ranges from 0 to 6 percent, according to published data. On average, the body weights of both male and female vegetarians are 3 percent to 20 percent lower than those of omnivores. Studies also have found that switching to a low-fat vegan diet leads to weight loss, even without changes to exercise or limits on portion sizes, calories, or carbohydrates. Finally, studies have found an increased calorie burn after vegan meals, meaning plant-based foods are being used more efficiently as fuel for the body, as opposed to being stored as fat.

If you're not interested in becoming vegetarian or vegan, that's fine, but I do believe that eating more plant-based meals per week is essential for pumping up your nutrient intake and getting better weight-loss results. A study of Seventh-Day Adventists, about 30 percent of whom follow a meatless diet, found that vegetarianism was associated with lower body mass indexes (BMIs). Within the thirty-four-thousand-plus population studied, BMI increased as the frequency of meat consumption increased, in both men and women. A study published in the *American Journal of Clinical Nutrition* compared six thousand vegetarians and five thousand nonvegetarians and found that BMI values were higher in nonvegetarians in all age groups for both genders. In addition, weight gain over a five-year period was lowest among people who adopted a diet containing fewer animal foods. In an Oxford University study that looked at nearly thirty-eight thousand adults, meat eaters had the highest BMIs for their age and vegans the lowest, with vegetarians and semivegetarians having intermediate values.

These studies were observational, meaning they simply looked at rates of overweight and obesity and correlated them with the subjects' diets. In an intervention study published in *Obesity,* researchers from the University of North Carolina at Chapel Hill looked at the effects on weight loss of a low-fat, vegan diet compared with a heart-healthy omnivore diet. Sixty-two overweight, postmenopausal women were randomly assigned to one of the two diets for fourteen weeks. The researchers found that individuals in the vegan group lost more weight than those in the omnivore group after both one year and two years. The differences were about eleven pounds versus four pounds in year one and about seven pounds versus two pounds in year two.

In a similar intervention, published in the *American Journal of Medicine,* researchers from George Washington University School of Medicine looked at how a low-fat, plant-based diet impacted body weight and metabolism, without a change in exercise, in free-living individuals. Sixty-four overweight, postmenopausal women were randomly assigned to a low-fat vegan diet or a heart-healthy omnivore diet. They weren't asked to limit their calorie intake and were told to not change their exercise programs. After fourteen weeks, the vegans had an average weight loss of thirteen pounds, compared with seven pounds in the omnivore group. Vegans also had higher rates of calorie burning, even at rest.

Vegetarians and vegans are often stereotyped as looking pale, sickly, and weak, but that hardly has been my experience. Quite the opposite: most are strong, energetic, and fit. Both vegans and omnivores can have nutrient-deficient diets: quality and balance are what matters.

**Bottom-Line Logic:** Vegetarians and semivegetarians often weigh less than omnivores, and eating more plant-based meals has been shown to control body weight even without a reduction in calories. Going veggie more often is an effective weight-loss tool.

## why: organic foods can boost your weight-loss results

There is no doubt that organic food is better for the environment, but it's also better for you, and going organic more often can also help you lose more weight, for two important reasons: (1) organic produce is higher

I am so happy with my results! Cynthia—you are a genius! I am still amazed at the amount of chocolate that I ate and the amount of weight I lost! Genius!

JESSICA, AGE 32

in antioxidants, as I discuss in chapter 2 (see page 74), and is linked to a boost in satiety and lower body weight, even without a reduction in calories; and (2) research shows that pesticide residues from conventionally grown foods may be a factor in mounting obesity rates.

A 2009 report by the French Agency for Food Safety found that organic foods—including fruits, vegetables, grains, meat, and dairy—contain more minerals and antioxidants, more "good" fats, and far fewer nitrates, which have been linked to a range of health problems, including diabetes and Alzheimer's, than nonorganic foods. New research shows that rats fed an organic diet sleep better, have stronger immune systems, and are slimmer than conventionally fed rodents. The combination of an abundance of satiating nutrients in organic food and a lack of chemicals may be the cause. Forty-three percent of organic-food buyers cite "better taste" as a major reason for purchasing organic fruits and vegetables.

In a study published in *Neurotoxicology and Teratology,* scientists found that rats exposed to pesticides gained considerable amounts of weight, and further research has linked pesticide exposure to a disruption of the endocrine system, which can trigger an increase in fat storage. Currently, a list of seventy-three pesticides is being reviewed for endocrine-disrupting effects by the Environmental Protection Agency, and another twenty-seven pesticides are defined as known or suspected hormone disruptors by the European Union. In a nutshell, endocrine disruptors mimic natural hormones in the body, block the effects of hormones, or cause the endocrine system to over- or underproduce hormones, including those that impact body weight.

In a study published in *Reproductive Toxicology,* researchers from the University of Wisconsin revealed their findings on pregnant mice exposed to small levels of chlorpyrifos, or CPFs, late in pregnancy. CPFs are used on fruit trees, including apple and orange trees, as well as corn. The mice were injected with three different minute levels of CPF, and 60 and again 150 days after birth, their offspring were evaluated for learning abilities, including their ability to find food, how fast they could find it, and how well they remembered where it was. Their thyroid-hormone levels also were tested. Trace amounts of the pesticide at the lowest levels didn't impact the male mice, but they significantly reduced the females' thyroid function and their abilities to find food. These problems persisted into adulthood.

Right now, organic agriculture isn't subsidized by the U.S. government, so there's no financial incentive for farmers to grow organic goods, and those who do face the financial hardship of the added costs. This is part of the reason the U.S. supply of organics isn't meeting the demand. A 2009 report found that nearly half of U.S. organic handlers found ingredients in short supply. Although certified organic acreage has doubled in the country since 1997, organic-food sales have quintupled over the same period. That's one reason you see so many imported organic goods.

There are seven reasons I'm so gung-ho about organics:

1. Organics don't use synthetic pesticides, which contaminate our food and land. This has implications for human weight control and health. Also, organic farmers don't use artificial fertilizers, which have been linked to algae blooms and "dead zones" in our oceans, as well as the risk of Alzheimer's, diabetes, and Parkinson's in humans.

2. Organic foods are richer in nutrients. This means they improve satiety and naturally help regulate body weight. (For more information on this research, see page 74.) Plants produce antioxidants to protect themselves from pests like insects and to withstand harsh weather. When they're treated with chemicals such as pesticides, they don't need to produce as much of their own natural defenses, so the levels are lower.

3. Organic foods don't contain genetically modified organisms, or GMOs. These have been linked to allergies and environmental concerns. For a primer on GMOs, see page 53.

4. Organic foods are grown in more nutritious soil. The conventional agricultural practice of repeatedly producing one crop using

chemical fertilizers has taken a toll on our farmland. The loss of topsoil is estimated at a cost of $40 billion per year in the United States, according to scientists from Cornell University. The poorer-quality soil remaining is less nutrient dense and produces "watered down" versions of fruits, vegetables, and grains.

5. Organically produced animal foods come from animals that are not given hormones and antibiotics. Conventional animal-based agriculture has contributed to a greater use of both types of substances, which impact human and environmental health. Today, approximately 80 percent of all U.S. feedlot cattle are injected with hormones, and the average dairy cow, which produced about fifty-three hundred pounds of milk a year in 1950, now pumps out more than eighteen thousand pounds. Yikes!

6. Organic farming promotes broader biodiversity—in other words, a great variety of different species in the ecosystem. Compared with a conventional farm, about 30 percent more species live on an organic farm. Birds, butterflies, soil organisms, beetles, earthworms, spiders, plant life, and mammals are all affected by agriculture, and organic farms are thriving habitats that support a healthy ecosystem. A loss of biodiversity has been linked to increases in allergies and a possible loss of species that could potentially treat or even cure serious diseases like cancer. A recent study found that 70 percent of the "new chemical entities" introduced into pharmacies within the past fifteen years came from nature. Before modern industrialized agriculture, farms produced about 80,000 species of plants; today farmers rely on about 150.

7. Organic farms produce higher-quality, tastier food. The term *organoleptic* refers to the sensory properties of a particular food—its taste, appearance, color, aroma, size, firmness, feel in the mouth, and even sound (e.g., the "snap" of a string bean or the "crack" you hear when biting into a crisp apple). Several published studies have shown that organic versions of foods rank higher in organoleptic characteristics. One study compared apples from an organic farm

with those from a conventional orchard less than a kilometer away. Without knowing which was which, trained tasters rated the organic apples as 14 percent firmer and 15 percent tastier. The organic versions contained 19 percent higher levels of phenolic antioxidants. Animal studies have also shown that hens, rats, and mice given free access to both organic and conventionally grown foods prefer the organic ones.

**Bottom-Line Logic:** Organic food is richer in nutrients and antioxidants, is more flavorful and satiating, and decreases your exposure to chemicals that can negatively impact your metabolism.

## go organic without breaking the bank

I realize that organic foods are more expensive than conventional foods, but I truly believe they are worth the extra cost. When I pass over a conventional food for an organic version, I actually see it as a bargain, since organic foods are richer in nutrients and better protect my health and the health of the planet. In any case, there are smart ways to save on organics:

- If you can buy only some organic foods, prioritize. The most important foods to buy organic are those that you eat every day or often, like milk and eggs, maybe oatmeal, and leafy greens.
- To boost your nutrient intake and reduce your exposure to pesticides, try to buy organic versions of the fruits and veggies that have been shown to carry the highest residues: peaches, apples, sweet bell peppers, celery, nectarines, strawberries, cherries, kale, lettuce, and grapes. Other top priorities

24 25 26 27 28 29 30

Diet Coke and I broke up, and he is taking Splenda and Equal with him. ☺ I am taking the smaller pants and the chocolate chips with me! Thank you again— this has been amazing!
JESSICA, AGE 32

---

## where did all the mom-and-pop farms go?

"Big agriculture," or huge factory-style farms, have been putting small and midsize farmers out of business at an alarming rate. Between 1993 and 1997, about fifty midsize family farms went under every single day. Colossal nonorganic farms benefit the most from government subsidies and tax breaks, and they manufacture mass quantities of a narrow range of relatively cheap crops. For more information about how to turn this trend around, visit www.sustainabletable.org.

---

include carrots, pears, spinach, potatoes, green beans, and cucumbers.

- Look for in-season organic produce. Locally grown fruits and veggies are generally some of the best buys in your market.
- Check out the sales, but buy an item only if it is already on your shopping list.
- Look for organic store brands. Many stores now have their own organic lines. (Whole Foods 365 organic is an example, as well as Safeway's O line.)
- Use coupons. You can find as much as one dollar off many items in the store.
- Buy in bulk. Dried fruit and grains such as oats, brown rice, and quinoa are great bulk purchases. No packaging means lower cost, a saving that normally gets passed on to you.

To learn more about organics, visit www.organic.org and www .organiccenter.org.

## look for the green USDA organic seal

The little green symbol on food labels that says "USDA certified organic" means the food was grown without synthetic pesticides, bioengineered genes (GMOs), or petroleum- or sewage-sludge-based fertilizers. The symbol also means that organic meat and dairy products are from animals fed organic, vegetarian feed, provided access to the outdoors, and not treated with hormones or antibiotics.

The USDA has defined three categories for the labeling of organic products. Meeting the requirements for any of these allows for usage of the organic seal:

100 Percent Organic: Made with 100 percent organic ingredients

Organic: Made with at least 95 percent organic ingredients

Made with Organic Ingredients: Made with a minimum of 70 percent organic ingredients, with strict restrictions on the remaining 30 percent, including no GMOs

Products with less than 70 percent organic ingredients may list organically produced ingredients on the side panel of the package, but they may not make any organic claims on the front of the package.

## why: the right ratio of protein to carbohydrate matters

Several studies have shown that a slight boost in protein and a like reduction in carbohydrates improves satiety and blood-sugar control and increases calorie burning. A Harvard study that followed sixty overweight men and women for six months found that those who were randomly assigned to a diet with 25 percent of their total calories from protein lost twice as much weight (about twenty pounds) as those following a plan with 12 percent of their calories from protein. Another study, published in the *American Journal of Clinical Nutrition*, found greater satisfaction, less hunger, and more weight loss when protein was increased to 30 percent of total calories and carbohydrates accounted for just 50 percent. When University of Alabama at Birmingham scientists compared subjects who ate a breakfast that had a standard percentage of calories from carbohydrates (55 percent) with those whose meal had slightly less (43 percent of calories), they found that the moderate-carb group had less fluctuation in their blood-sugar levels and greater feelings of fullness in the hours after the meal.

In my practice, I've been increasingly encouraging clients who are less active or over forty to slightly curb their carbohydrate intakes. I don't recommend a diet that drastically restricts carbs, because that will severely limit your intake of antioxidants, fiber, vitamins, and minerals, as well as deprive your brain of its number one fuel source and wreak havoc with your mood. Not getting enough means those nutrients don't show up for work in your body day after day, which leads to less-than-optimal performance and health, and even an increased risk of the diseases these nutrients protect you from.

On the flip side, eating too many carbs overloads your body and leads to weight gain. I aim for a middle ground: 45 percent at the low end and 65 percent at the high end. For a 1,500-calorie diet, 45 percent is 169 grams of carbs and 65 percent is 244 grams; that's a pretty wide range.

**Bottom-Line Logic:** I have found that unless I'm working with a professional or endurance athlete, the best ratio of carbs, protein, and fat for weight management, blood-sugar control, and satiety tends to be about 45 to 50 percent carbs, 20 to 25 percent protein, and 30 to 35 percent fat.

This plan is based on these percentages. It reflects the way I eat every day and what I use with most of my clients to get results.

## why: processed foods affect your health and weight

It's pretty intuitive that processed foods aren't as healthy as fresh, whole foods, but a lot of people have asked me, "What's so bad about them, really?" Several recent studies have found that preservatives and excessive sodium are hardly the only problematic aspects of a processed diet.

In 2009, the U.S. nonprofit group Consumers Union (CU) tested packaged foods, including soups, juice, tuna, and green beans, and found that almost all contained measurable levels of bisphenol A, or BPA—a building block of plastics that's been linked to a host of health problems, including disrupted thyroid function and obesity. Scientists say BPA may act like estrogen in the body, and in the CU test BPA was found even in foods labeled as organic and BPA-free. BPA is known to leach into foods from containers and is therefore thought to be routinely ingested. One recent study detected BPA in 92.6 percent of the urine samples collected from a U.S. population. Animal studies have found that BPA accelerates the formation of fat cells. Exposure of in utero mice to low doses of BPA also led to weight gain, and female mice fed a low dose of BPA in their drinking water packed on 13 percent more body weight.

A study published in the *Journal of Clinical Endocrinology and Metabolism* found that compounds in packaged foods drive up inflammation and premature aging by introducing substances in our diets called advanced glycation end products, or AGEs. AGEs are toxic substances produced in abundance in American diets by "doing stuff" to fresh food, including heating, drying, smoking, or frying it. They're also formed when meats are grilled. These nasty compounds promote oxidation and inflammation in the body, which are triggers for premature aging and chronic diseases including diabetes, heart disease, and obesity. (For a

## more fiber, less belly fat

Eating just a little bit more fiber could have a big impact on trimming your waistline, according to research from the University of Southern California published in the *American Journal of Clinical Nutrition*. Scientists asked eighty-five overweight teens to fill out a questionnaire about their eating habits and then report on their diet again two years later. Belly fat increased 21 percent among those who were eating less fiber, but the young people who had upped their fiber intake had a 4 percent reduction in belly fat. Cinch! includes fiber-rich foods every day. Some of the best sources of fiber featured in the plan include bean-based dishes such as the California Sunshine Salad or Mediterranean Lentils over Couscous.

refresher on oxidation, see the box titled "Grapes, the Secret Berry," on page 105.)

Scientists from the U.S. National Institute on Aging and Mount Sinai School of Medicine reported that reducing the intake of AGEs is one of the simplest ways to improve overall health, even without changing your total calorie intake. They looked at forty people who were randomly assigned to one of two diets: one group continued to eat their typical American meals, and a second group ate a diet with the same overall calorie and nutrient content but with 50 percent fewer AGEs. After four months, blood AGE levels and markers for inflammation plummeted by as much as 60 percent in the intervention group.

Another study, published in *Environmental Health Perspectives,* suggests that polyfluoroalkyl chemicals, or PFCs, found in food packaging may boost blood cholesterol levels. PFCs are highly stable compounds that persist in the human body for more than eight years. Data from the National Health and Nutrition Examination Survey (NHANES) showed that PFCs were present in the bodies of nearly all the participants they studied. When scientists analyzed the relationship between blood concentrations of four types of PFCs and cholesterol, they found that people with levels in the top 25 percent had higher total and non-HDL cholesterol (primarily LDL, or "bad," cholesterol) than those who scored in the lowest 25 percent.

Finally, eating a diet high in processed foods has been linked to an increased risk of depression, according to British research published in the *British Journal of Psychiatry*. Scientists collected data on the diets of thirty-five hundred middle-aged civil servants and looked at depression rates five years later. They split the participants into two diet categories: those who ate a diet largely based on whole foods, and those who ate a mainly processed-foods diet. After accounting for factors including gender, age, education, physical activity, smoking habits, and chronic diseases, they found a significant difference. Those who ate the most whole foods had a 26 percent lower risk of future depression compared with those who ate the least, and people with a diet high in processed food had a 58 percent higher risk of depression than those who ate few processed products.

**Bottom-Line Logic:** The best way to avoid BPA, PFCs, and other artificial and chemical additives is to eat more fresh, whole foods. In an ideal world, none of our food would come from a box, can, bag, bottle, or jar, but I know that's not realistic. I've limited the packaged foods in this plan, and when you're at the market, keep these tips in mind:

- Cut back on packaging wherever you can. Buy in bulk, and instead of purchasing products like a plastic bottle of lime juice, opt for freshly squeezed wedges.
- For packaged foods with more than one ingredient, like corn tortillas and chocolate chips, buy only brands made with ingredients you can clearly recognize and pronounce and would use in your

own kitchen. The ingredient list is always the very first thing you should look for on a label. If the list reads like a recipe, you're in business. If it sounds like a science experiment rather than food, consider another option. In my opinion, store-bought bread should include only whole grains, water, yeast, and salt—that's all.

# 8

`24 25 26 27 28 29 30 31 32 33`

# conquer emotional eating

Most of us developed an emotional relationship with food as children. We were comforted, consoled, lulled, rewarded, even babysat with food—a lollipop at the scary doctor's office, a bowl of sugary cereal and cartoons so mom could talk on the phone in peace, a dish of ice cream after a teasing incident at school, a pizza party for an especially good report card, warm cookies and milk after waking up from a bad dream. From a really young age, you probably learned to turn to food as a companion or coping mechanism for just about every feeling, from fear to joy.

As human beings, we don't like to feel negative emotions, and food is an effective and powerful way to detach, distract yourself from uncomfortable feelings, or stuff them down so you don't have to experience them. On the flip side, the pleasure food brings can also amplify feelings of happiness when you eat in celebration. In a nutshell, emotional eating works!

I struggled all my life with weight. It is such a sore topic for me. I am very hard on myself. Having two kids really put me over the top. I have struggled for so long, thinking I just had no willpower. Now I see everything I was doing wrong. It just puts a lump in my throat.

LAURENE, AGE 36

Both psychologically and biologically, eating, even when you're not hungry, feels good in the moment. Unfortunately, that fleeting feeling is often followed by guilt, regret, weight gain (or stalled weight loss), and possibly the aggravation of health problems like gastric reflux and high blood pressure. But in my experience, the problems generated by emotional eating may not be enough to stop you from turning to Ben & Jerry's. Over the years I've counseled countless people who wanted nothing more than to stop using food to meet their emotional needs, but they just couldn't seem to do it, even with their health on the line or an important event looming, such as their own wedding. Why couldn't they stop? In this chapter I'll reveal what I shared with them, and help you learn how to break the cycle.

You don't have to complete all the exercises in this chapter right away. Start by reading through the pages, and at some point during Cinch!, commit to going back and working through the exercises at your own pace. Sometimes emotional eating isn't obvious, and it doesn't mean that you have deep psychological issues that require therapy. But it's important to explore what role emotional eating may play in your life. I have included a number of tools to help you tease out your specific issues. If emotional eating turns out to be one of the greatest hurdles in your ability to successfully change your relationship with food, I believe the information and resources in the chapter will help you begin to break the cycle.

Emotional eating is socially acceptable in the United States, even socially reinforced by our families, our peers, the media, and advertisements. I used to collect ads that reinforced emotional eating to use when teaching about emotional eating. Nearly every week, I'd come across a new example, typically with copy that read something like, "Go ahead,"

"Give in," and "You deserve it." Constant reminders that food feels good are one of the many reasons it's difficult to stop using food as a substitute for something else. But if you really get to the root of what food "gives" you and then fill that need in another way, even the most enticing ad campaign or frustratingly bad day won't trigger an eating incident.

## understanding your food/feelings connections

Psychologists say that every emotion is rooted in one of four primary categories: fear, sadness, anger, and joy. Feeling anxious and feeling overwhelmed are essentially forms of fear; loneliness is tied to sadness, and frustration to anger. To learn more about your food/feelings connections, try this exercise: Take out a sheet of paper and make four columns, one for each primary emotion. In each column, note a recent or significant incident that elicited that particular feeling. Now, think back to the day of the event, and try to remember whether you ate in response.

For example, when one of my clients filled out this table, she realized that the anger she felt about how she had been treated by her boss led her to add to her cart at the drugstore a bag of Twizzlers, which she immediately opened in the parking lot and ate during her drive home. Another client realized that the sadness she felt about being away from home during the holidays was probably why she baked brownies, a major comfort food, and ate half the pan while she watched *Elf* (again).

When these things are happening, it's not always obvious why. Many of my clients think that incidents like this are about not having enough willpower, but nothing could be further from the truth. You probably don't think, "I'm angry, so I'm going to gnaw on some licorice or tear into a pizza." It just sort of happens. But connecting the dots between your feelings and behavior is the foundation of being able to change. And the first step is awareness.

Building awareness is like stumbling around in a dark room, and then finding the dimmer switch and slowly turning it up until the entire space is illuminated and you can see everything in detail. It generally happens in steps or stages.

When you first start to build awareness, you may realize that you ate emotionally only after the fact, maybe as you toss the empty carton of ice cream into the trash. The next step is to catch yourself during the act. As you bite into a potato chip you may stop and think, "What am I doing? Why am I eating this?" Then eventually it hits you as you reach for food: you realize that you're standing in front of the fridge with the door open not because your body needs fuel, but because your mind needs a diversion.

When you get to this point—which will be before you know it by using the exercises in this chapter—you'll be at a significant crossroads. If you go ahead and eat, you'll be doing so with full awareness. In other words, you'll be making a conscious choice to eat emotionally. Even if you proceed, it will be an entirely different experience than doing it mindlessly.

One of my clients realized this while she was in line at a fast-food drive-through. With cars in front of and behind her, she couldn't get out of line, but when it struck her that she ended up there because she was mad at her husband (and not the least bit hungry), the idea of escaping in a crispy chicken sandwich and fries felt a lot less appealing. So she ordered the sandwich without the fries, pulled into a parking spot, and unwrapped it. As she took a bite, it hit her that this wasn't really what she needed, and suddenly she was fully aware of the grease and salt coating her mouth. Disgusted, she tossed the sandwich back in the bag.

This moment was a major revelation and turning point in her relationship with food. In the past, a fast-food meal, which she barely tasted and often ate while driving as her mind raced, allowed her to push her feelings down. Food served as a brief reprieve that helped her get through the rest of the day. But understanding what she was doing as it was happening brought her to an entirely new place. She realized that she didn't *need* fast food; she needed to address her feelings. Her mission was to

---

## individualized help

This chapter is by no means meant to be a substitute for therapy. If you feel that you would benefit from one-on-one counseling, check with your insurance provider about how to contact a therapist in your area, or, to find a local licensed psychologist, visit http://locator.apa.org. This chapter is designed to help you identify emotional eating, find healthy alternatives, and learn to eat in response to physical, rather than emotional, cues. A therapist's role is much deeper. He or she can help you work through your feelings and address the circumstances that may be their wellspring, such as an unhappy relationship, self-esteem issues, unresolved family issues, or significant events in your past.

---

find other ways to do so that were just as effective, but also self-nurturing and healthy.

That last part is key, because if food is meeting an emotional need and you take it away without putting something else in its place, it's like pulling the rug out from under yourself. You're going to stumble, and either you'll wind up right back where you started or, to fill the gap, you'll switch to another coping mechanism, one that may be just as unhealthy. I once had a client who decided that a gastric-bypass operation was her best option. Postsurgery, she was no longer able to eat emotionally without becoming physically ill, so she unconsciously began using shopping as a substitute for food. Within six months she had maxed out two credit cards. That's when she realized that over all those years, she didn't have a problem with food; she had a problem with not acknowledging her feelings and addressing them in a healthier way.

In many cases, you can't change the situation that led to the emotions you're experiencing, such as a job you can't quit today or a family member who is ill, but you can change your awareness of those emotions and your reaction to the situation. I call one of the tools I share with my clients *mind mapping*. It involves tracking or linking a specific situation to your feelings and subsequent behavior.

Here's how to get started: Over the next week, select a time to "take inventory" once a day, maybe just after you get in bed, when you're relaxed and not distracted. Think through the events of the day, from the time you woke up to the time you got under the covers. Run through the four major emotions: fear, sadness, anger, and joy. On a scale from zero to ten, how intensely did any of the day's happenings spark these feelings? (A zero represents no response in that category; ten, a powerful sense of that emotion.)

Now reflect on your food choices for the day. Do you see any patterns? The more focused time you spend each day thinking through these connections, the more awareness you'll develop in the moment, just like my client at the drive-through. She trashed that chicken sandwich not because she "shouldn't" eat it and not because it didn't fit into the rules of this diet, but because her awareness allowed her to see that she didn't need it and it no longer felt right.

## finding alternatives to food that really work

For the next few moments, take a visual journey with me. Imagine being in a clearing of some kind—maybe an open field, beach, or valley. Ahead you see a beautiful tent that draws you toward it. On the flap you see a sign that reads: ONCE YOU ENTER THIS TENT, NO ONE WILL BE ABLE TO OBSERVE OR INTERRUPT YOU. TAKE AS MUCH TIME AS YOU NEED.

As you enter, every food you've ever known of fills the space—every restaurant or grocery item, every meal you've had on vacation, every homemade family recipe—and it's all in unlimited quantities. In other words, if you take an ice-cream sundae, another one will pop up in its place. Take a few moments to look around. Now, answer these two questions:

1. How do you feel about being in this space?
2. What do you want to do?

Your responses will tell you a lot about your relationship with food. In chapter 2, I explain that you were born with an inherent desire to take care of yourself and feel good, which becomes stifled during your toddler years. As a baby, your desire to eat is driven by the physical need for food and to feel good. Babies aren't aware of splurge foods or comfort foods, and babies don't eat emotionally. Babies essentially have twenty-four-hour access to food, but they choose to start and stop eating according to what feels best physically.

If your response to question one involved an emotion, maybe fear or joy, food has likely been serving a role in your life that goes beyond nourishing you. That doesn't mean you shouldn't have any emotional ties to food. It's normal to enjoy a delicious meal. But when the eating is initiated solely by emotions, without regard to what your body needs or what would feel best physically, the food/feelings relationship has tipped out of balance. If you wrote "afraid" for question one, maybe you feel as if you can't trust yourself around food, that if you don't restrict yourself you'll binge out of control. Or maybe you wrote "excited" in anticipation of indulging. Whatever your response, ask yourself: Does it feel natural, the way a baby would react? Or does it feel like something I learned? If you learned this response, how and where was it passed on? (More on this to come.)

For question two, if you didn't feel any strong emotions, you probably didn't want to eat—unless you had physical symptoms of hunger. If you weren't emotional or hungry, you may have wanted to explore and look around out of curiosity, but you probably wouldn't dive in. That's because, as I discussed in chapter 2, eating when you're not physically hungry doesn't feel good, and eating beyond the point of being full and satisfied doesn't feel good, just as it doesn't feel good to not eat when you are physically hungry.

The point of this exercise is to see that emotional eaters decide whether, when, what, and how much to eat based on their feelings. Overcoming emotional eating means that you'll be able to rely on your physi-

# MY STORY

### Jennifer Steinruck, 37  |  Pounds lost in 5 days: 7

## I Lost 1.5 Inches from My Waist in 5 Days!

I wanted to try the Fast Forward because my weight had spiraled up over the last several years. A divorce, four kids, and my busy work schedule led me to processed and fast food. Before I started the plan my portions were much too large and I ate too quickly and too often. If I felt the slightest bit hungry, I would eat anything. I ate when I was bored or stressed and paid no attention to the time I ate or what foods I chose. I used artificial sweeteners in my coffee and tea and drank sugary beverages loaded with empty calories.

My kids were following my example, and I knew I had to make some drastic changes. When Cynthia gave me the details of the plan, it was just what I needed to get back on track to a healthier, happier family.

My first Fast Forward meal, the scramble, was easy to prepare and very good. The parfait was good, too. I was pleasantly surprised at the taste of the yogurt. It reminded me of sour cream, which I like, and the almonds added a crunch. That night I ate dinner, the salad, poolside with friends. I was at a huge

cal sensations of hunger and eat in a way that best supports a feeling of wellness, just like a baby. The goal is to simultaneously feel full but not overly full—satisfied, energized, and ready to move on with your day.

To help you learn more about your food/feelings connections, I put together the following series of exercises. I know the questions are not easy to answer, but you don't have to write in your response right away. Think them through, even for several days, to see what surfaces.

buffet stocked with many foods and drinks I like, so I was really glad that the salad was so tasty. Several people commented on how good my meal looked!

On day two I felt really good at breakfast. I was able to sit with my family and enjoy my meal, which is a treat by itself. I was surprised that my "small" portions were able to satisfy me. Normally I would have grabbed just anything.

On day three I was feeling really good about following the plan despite so many temptations. I managed to avoid all my common pitfalls simply by thinking ahead and carrying a cooler. Even in the evenings I stayed on track. Once the kids are tucked into bed, I tend to "reward" myself with poor snack choices. But I realized that by picking the right foods and watching the time, I can avoid boredom binging and stress eating.

The Fast Forward was a real eye-opener for me. In just a few days I learned to recognize what my body had been trying to tell me for a long time. I'm ecstatic about my results. I wasn't expecting to lose seven pounds and inches off my waist in just days!

Before Cinch! I had no idea what a realistic portion size was. This plan gave me the information and motivation to move forward making positive choices that will affect my entire family. My pantry is now stocked with healthy food, and when I go out to dinner with friends I look at the menu ahead of time so I won't be caught off guard.

Complete this Food and Feelings grid:

|  | Fear | Sadness | Anger | Joy |
|---|---|---|---|---|
| When I'm experiencing this emotion, food makes me feel (fill in the box). |  |  |  |  |
| What healthy behaviors, aside from eating, have I tried that allow me to avoid this emotion (e.g., not drinking alcohol, shopping, gambling, etc.)? |  |  |  |  |
| What other behaviors would I like to try that may allow me to address this feeling? |  |  |  |  |

One you've identified some healthy alternatives to eating, you can begin to test them. It's very much a trial-and-error process, and there are a few important things to keep in mind. First, doing something different may feel awkward in the beginning, but the more you try it, the more natural it will feel. For example, one of my clients became aware enough to stop herself *before* using food, but at first, she said, it felt weird for her to do a deep-breathing exercise instead; thoughts of food kept popping into her head. But the more she stuck with the breathing and tried other

Sample response:

| | Fear | Sadness | Anger | Joy |
|---|---|---|---|---|
| When I'm experiencing this emotion, food makes me feel (fill in the box). | Less anxious, numb, detached | Comforted, almost like being given a hug, sometimes detached or numb | A sense of release, cutting loose, rebellious | Carefree, rewarded |
| What behaviors, aside from eating, have I tried that allow me to avoid this emotion (e.g., not drinking alcohol, shopping, gambling, etc.)? | Deep breathing, talking to someone I trust | Crying, taking a hot shower or bath, drinking a cup of tea while I read, spending time with my pets or children | Walking fast, gardening (pulling up weeds, tilling soil), cleaning, anything physical | Singing, getting a chair massage, watching one of my favorite happy movies, like *Grease* or *The Wizard of Oz* |
| What other behaviors would I like to try that may allow me to address this feeling? | Meditating, starting a hobby that takes my mind off things, like photography, knitting, or sewing | Writing, connecting with other people, maybe volunteering with people in need, getting out in nature, maybe a community garden | Dancing, playing an instrument like keyboards, yoga | Painting or drawing, something creative |

things, such as writing in a journal and making jewelry, the more she found that cookies were no longer her first thought.

To successfully employ an alternative, you need to "catch" the emotion before it becomes too intense. Think of an intensity spectrum from zero to ten, with zero indicating no sense of the emotion and ten indicating maxi-

## sadness outeats happiness

When Cornell University scientists recruited volunteers to eat grapes and popcorn while watching either a funny movie (*Sweet Home Alabama*) or a sad, depressing flick (*Love Story*), they found a significant difference. Those who watched the sad movie ate 36 percent more popcorn than those who saw the upbeat film. The *Sweet Home Alabama* group ate both popcorn and grapes, but they spent much more time popping grapes as they laughed through the movie. The researchers concluded that happy people want to maintain or extend their mood, and at least subconsciously, they tend to consider the long term; as such, they choose foods with more nutritional value. People who feel sad, on the other hand, choose more indulgent, tasty snacks that give them a feeling of instant gratification.

mum strength. By the time you've reached a six or a seven, it may be much more difficult, if not impossible, to stop yourself and try an alternative. For that reason, it helps to be able to scope out your emotions. Think about your body. It always prefers a perfect balance, which is why it tries to tell you when something doesn't feel right. When you're dehydrated, you get thirsty; too warm, you sweat and feel flushed; too cold, you shiver and get goose bumps; too tired, you yawn, your head nods, and you have trouble keeping your eyes open. Emotions have symptoms, too.

Symptoms of fear may include:

- Tightness in your chest or throat
- Oversensitivity to noise
- Breathlessness
- Muscle weakness
- Lack of energy
- Butterflies in your stomach

- Sighing
- Sleep disturbances
- Appetite disturbances
- Absentmindedness
- Social withdrawal
- Restlessness

Symptoms of sadness may include:

- Inability to focus
- Heaviness in your chest
- Lack of energy
- Appetite changes
- Sleep disorders
- Crying
- Feeling blue or down
- Not enjoying your usual activities or hobbies
- Social withdrawal
- Pessimism

Symptoms of anger may include:

- Feeling hot and flushed
- Hairs standing up
- Hyperactivity
- Racing heartbeat
- Tension in your arms, neck, or shoulders
- Headache
- Swearing
- Agitation
- Deriving satisfaction from other people's problems
- Negative self-talk
- Confrontations with others

Symptoms of joy may include:

- Feeling "illuminated"
- Using a soft, expressive tone of voice
- Feeling agile and "light" in your movements
- Enthusiasm
- Glimmering eyes
- Smiling
- Talking with and complimenting others more than usual

## unlearning emotional eating

When a behavior has been reinforced for decades, undoing it overnight isn't a realistic goal. But the more you explore, the easier it is to untangle your feelings from your eating habits. Here's another exercise that may help.

Complete this Digging Deeper grid:

|  | Fear | Sadness | Anger | Joy |
|---|---|---|---|---|
| When or how did I learn to use food to cope with this emotion? |  |  |  |  |
| What problems has turning to food to cope with my feelings caused for me? |  |  |  |  |

| | Fear | Sadness | Anger | Joy |
|---|---|---|---|---|
| On a scale from 0 to 10, how confident do I feel about my ability to try alternatives to eating (0 indicates no confidence; 10, maximum confidence)? | | | | |
| If my confidence level is a 5 or below, what might help me feel more confident? | | | | |
| To whom can I turn for support? | | | | |
| What changes could make my home or workplace more supportive? | | | | |

I know that as much as you want to lose weight and improve your health, it can feel overwhelming. In some ways, learning a new way of relating to food is like learning to speak a new language, and if you have a history of emotional eating, it can be even more challenging. So if meal planning doesn't come completely naturally right away, please don't beat yourself up. I promise: it will get easier every day. And before you know it, this will become your usual way of eating. In fact, eventually it will feel so natural and normal that you'll barely have to think about it. But it does take practice.

While writing this book, I decided to learn how to play the guitar. I'd been wanting to play for years, but I kept putting it off. When my birthday rolled around, I finally decided that this would be the year, so I bought a guitar and signed up for my first ten-week class. The first two weeks were incredible. It was new and exciting, and as I walked to class with my guitar case strapped to my back, I felt so proud of myself. By week four I started to have doubts. The lessons were getting more complicated, and though I practiced daily and did my "homework," it wasn't exactly coming naturally. One night after class I was feeling overwhelmed, frustrated, and disappointed in myself, and to be honest, a part of me wanted to quit. I was venting to a friend, and she said, "Cynthia, you've only had five one-hour classes. You're just getting started. Don't be so hard on yourself!" As soon as she said that, I actually burst out laughing, because she was telling me the exact same thing I say to my clients.

As humans, we're programmed to resist change. Anything that's new and different feels weird and challenging in the beginning, but I'm 100 percent sure that you have conquered many learning curves in your life and mastered skills that seemed overwhelming in the beginning but eventually became second nature. You've probably learned how to swim, ride a bike, drive a car, and many other things—from work-related expertise to using an iPhone. Every time you feel even a slight glimmer of self-doubt, take a moment and think about what you've mastered. Here are five more tips to help you along the way:

**1. Say No to Yesism.** *Yesism* is actually a textbook term defined as the inability to say no. Not being able to set boundaries can lead you to feeling overwhelmed and trigger you to turn to food as an outlet. If you chronically take on too much, set a goal of politely saying no the next time you're asked to take on any additional responsibilities.

**2. Take Mini Mental Vacations.** If on the spectrum of emotional intensity you begin to reach a tipping point and your thoughts turn toward food, try this visualization exercise: Close your eyes and take yourself to a relaxing place you've been before. It could be a past vacation spot, the park where you walk your dog, or even the couch in your living room or your bed. As you look around in your mind, take in the colors, textures, even smells of this relaxing spot. Immerse yourself in this environment for just a few minutes. You can do this anytime, anyplace, and just visualizing a calming environment can quickly help you manage your emotions and avoid a spontaneous eating episode.

**3. Check Your Self-Talk.** We all talk to ourselves in our heads, and too often that chatter is self-deprecating. As I mentioned in chapter 2, in workshops, I've asked women to say exactly what they're thinking while looking in a mirror. They typically don't want to, partly because it's private, and partly because saying it seems more harsh than thinking it. But facing those thoughts is important, because even though they are unspoken, they deeply affect how you feel. Negative self-talk leads to negative emotions such as anger and sadness and causes you to want to cope by using food. If you catch yourself being nasty to yourself in your mind, stop and ask yourself, "Would I say that out loud to my best friend?" Focus on treating yourself, including how you talk to yourself, like you would treat the person you love and care about the most.

> One of the best things that I have learned from this plan is to set a structure to the times I eat. I really feel that I am eating more than before—and the foods are healthier!
>
> JESSICA, AGE 32

**4. Ask for Support.** A lack of support from your family members, co-workers, and friends can make changing your relationship with food ten times more challenging. Even those you're closest to may underestimate how serious you are, or fail to understand how important this is to you. If they're not on board, gently remind them of something in their lives that required your support, and ask for theirs in return.

**5. Do Something Just for You.** Some emotional eaters say that indulging in food is the only thing they have that makes them feel good or is just for them. A lack of fulfillment in your life can create a gap that food fills, but only in the moment. Commit to carving out some just-for-you time, whether it's to express your creativity, to relax, or simply to be silly and have fun. Fueling your spirit can help you change an unhealthy relationship with food.

## the chocolate-chip exercise

Sometimes my new clients expect me to be the food police, but I'm not that kind of nutritionist. In addition to my degrees in nutrition science, I completed formal training in counseling and health education. I've also worked in inpatient eating-disorder treatment centers, and I work closely with mental-health professionals.

Because I come from a "whole person" perspective (physical, emotional, social, occupational, intellectual, spiritual, and environmental), my clients get very "real" with me about their eating behaviors. Many of them have talked about feeling so compelled to eat that they took food out of the garbage or secretly ate in a bathroom stall. I never judge my clients' deepest, darkest secrets about eating. Instead, I try to help them understand and escape the turmoil. As I've said, raising awareness is key, so I have created a ten-step exercise that can really raise your consciousness about the pace and experience of eating. Here's how it works:

1. Choose a quiet time when you won't be interrupted, and turn off any distractions, such as the television or your MP3 player.
2. Place ten chocolate chips on a small plate or napkin.
3. Sit upright in a chair at your dining table, with the chips in front of you.
4. Close your eyes.
5. Very slowly take a deep breath in through your nose, and when your lungs are full, hold the breath for a count of one, and slowly release it through your mouth.
6. Repeat the previous step five times. With each repetition, draw all of your energy and attention to your breathing. With each breath out, imagine your thoughts and distractions being blown away so you can simply focus on your breathing in this moment.
7. With a straight back, slowly and gently lift your shoulders toward your ears as you breathe in. When you've raised them as high as

possible, hold for a count of one, and slowly relax them as you breathe out, returning to your original position. Repeat this procedure three times, and each time you release your shoulders, let go of any tension trapped in your muscles.

8. Now take one chip and put it in your mouth. Do not chew it. Allow the chip to melt on your tongue, and draw all of your energy and attention to the flavor, texture, taste, and feel of the chocolate.

9. When the first chip has melted, take another. Again, let it melt, and savor every morsel. Repeat until the chips are gone.

10. Take out a piece of paper or a journal, and write down your thoughts and reactions.

After completing this exercise, most of my clients will say things like, "That was the best chocolate I ever tasted," "I can't believe how long it took me to eat ten chocolate chips," and "Wow, that was intense." Very few people have ever experienced eating in this incredibly focused, deliberate way. One of my clients said, "I usually throw a small handful of chocolate chips in my mouth and chew them while I start getting dinner ready or grab the laundry out of the dryer. I never thought about what it would be like to eat them one at a time."

Completing the exercise even once can open you up to an entirely new way of experiencing food. It can help you learn to catch yourself eating too fast or eating without any awareness of the taste, flavor, texture, and mouth feel of what you're eating.

One of my clients who was single and lived alone had a nightly routine of going home from work, making her standard dinner (whole-wheat pasta with tomato sauce, veggies, and chicken), and eating it in front of the TV while she watched *Jeopardy*. For her, eating a healthy dinner wasn't the problem. She basically ate the same fairly nutritious meal night after night. But a few hours after dinner she'd find herself rummaging through her cupboards and munching on anything, from stale crackers to a handful of cereal.

A few days after the Chocolate-Chip Exercise, she had a revelation.

She said, "As I was eating, it hit me that I was wolfing down my food and not really tasting it. So I stopped, turned off the TV, went in the kitchen, took a few deep breaths, and kept eating—and guess what? I realized that I didn't want to be eating pasta. I wanted something cold and crunchy. So I put my dinner down the garbage disposal and went to the grocery store!"

She went on to describe how different this shopping experience was from her typical trip to the supermarket. Instead of tossing her predictable items in the cart, she felt like a kid in a candy store. She said, "I

## how your relationship impacts your weight and emotions

Once you say, "I do," both partners tend to pack on the pounds. A Cornell University study published in the journal *Social Science and Medicine* found that newlyweds gain more weight on average than singles or people who are widowed or divorced (although women tend to gain more weight in the first year of marriage than men do). Another study, in *Obesity Research,* found that on average, married people gain six to eight pounds over a two-year period. And if the relationship isn't blissful, it gets worse for women. One study found that among twenty-five thousand married women, those who claimed to be in an unhappy relationship gained an average of fifty-four pounds during the first ten years of marriage.

If you're married, your spouse can be one of the greatest influences on what, when, and how much you eat, because couples eat together more often than they jointly partake in just about any other activity. You may be lucky enough to have separate closets or bathrooms, but chances are you'll share one kitchen—and when your foods are under the same roof, the potential for food fights and weight gain skyrockets. The following five tips can help you avoid both:

1. Have "me," "you," and "us" food spaces. Chances are, you and your partner are going to have different food preferences, and some of his

may be foods you prefer to avoid, from bloody raw meat that grosses you out to salt-and-vinegar chips you can't resist diving into. Create separate areas in the fridge, freezer, and cupboards for each of your foods, and a common area for foods you share. Out-of-sight, out-of-mind goes a long way toward preventing arguments (e.g., "Your meat juices dripped on my spinach!") and temptations (if those chips are the first thing you see when you open the cabinet, chances are, you'll be polishing them off). Men and women nearly always separate their bathroom toiletries; doing the same in the kitchen just makes sense.

2. Agree to a no-food-gifts policy. Food is a powerful and intimate connector, but bringing each other food favorites as a sign of affection can lead to major weight gain and health problems. Tell each other the nonfood ways you love to be loved. I've told my husband, Jack, that back rubs and handwritten notes are at the top of my list.

3. Squelch eating as entertainment. After tying the knot, a lot of couples start going out less in favor of ordering pizzas and Netflix films or grilling at home. Or they start doing fewer "date nights" on the weekends (like going to a concert or comedy club) and engaging in more food-focused activities like going to brunch. Try to keep your social life active, and when you're deciding what to do, make food secondary and not the main attraction.

4. Never "split" a dish evenly. Even at the same height, men burn about 20 percent more calories than women at rest because they carry more muscle mass. And because men are typically taller, the calorie divide gets even wider. Bottom line: men and women's metabolisms are like SUVs versus compact cars. It's best to customize your meals to your body's calorie-burning engine. For directions on how to tailor this plan to your body's needs or your spouse's, see page 154.

5. If you feel a food conflict brewing (you disagree about how to feed your new puppy, you're never hungry at the same time, he pushes food on you after you've said no . . . ), talk about it right away. Ignoring it can result in resentment that affects the quality of your relationship. Bring the issue up at a quiet time when you can talk it through, and use nonaccusatory language like "Can I talk to you about something? I've noticed that . . ." instead of "It really bothers me when you . . ."

thought to myself: I can buy and make anything I want!" and exploring her options began to feel like a new adventure. She decided on romaine, red onions, carrots, fresh basil, and sunflower seeds to satisfy her cold crunchy craving. She bought frozen precooked shrimp and frozen corn, which she thawed to top her salad, and she splurged on a somewhat expensive bottle of fig-infused vinegar. Her meal perfectly fit the Cinch! 5-Piece Puzzle.

She reported feeling completely satisfied at the end of her meal, and it was the first night in months that her thoughts didn't turn to food in the evening. In fact, when she was brushing her teeth before bed, she realized that when she went into the kitchen to feed her dog, she didn't even think about doing any postdinner nibbling. She also had a newfound sense of excitement about meal planning.

Though it wasn't obvious to my client, she and I discovered that emotionally, her pattern was rooted in sadness. She was single and living alone, and subconsciously she just wanted to get dinner over with because she was cooking only for herself. Robotically preparing the same standard meal night after night allowed her to remain detached from her feelings about wanting to be in a relationship. But the enthusiasm she discovered for exploring new foods transformed her social life. She started shopping at ethnic, local, and gourmet markets she never knew about, having friends over for dinner—and, yes, she began meeting other singles!

# 9

24 25 26 27 28 29 30 31 32 33

# fall in love with walking

C an you lose weight without exercising? It's a question I hear often, and the answer, truthfully, is yes. And yet I consider exercise a crucial part of the Cinch! plan. That's because research shows, and my experience confirms, that exercise is important for speeding up weight loss and keeping the weight off. In fact, 90 percent of successful "losers"—people who have lost more than thirty pounds and kept it off for years—exercise on a daily basis.

If you already work out for at least thirty minutes five days a week, rock on! Keep doing what you're doing. I have included this chapter for anyone who struggles to be consistently active or has a hard time mustering up the motivation to get moving. If you are one of those people—and 60 percent of Americans are in that group, according to the Centers for Disease Control and Prevention—I want to help you get started by falling in love with walking.

Brisk walking on a regular basis can do wonders for your mind, body, and spirit. In addition to helping you lose weight faster by torching additional calories, walking will do amazing things for your health, such as reducing your blood pressure and lowering your risk of developing breast cancer and diabetes. Walking also pumps out endorphins, the feel-good chemicals linked to "runner's high," and boosts your stamina and body satisfaction, even without weight loss. Have you ever started your day feeling pretty good about yourself, and then a single event, like trying on a dress that is too tight, sends your body image tumbling? An exhilarating walk can turn your day back around. If you're still not convinced to lace up your walking shoes, read "Six More Reasons to Get Moving," on page 237, and the section of this chapter titled, "The Four Unique Benefits of Walking."

I don't recommend doing any exercise during the Fast Forward. But if you've been inactive or inconsistently active, I do ask you to commit to starting a walking program by day seven of the Cinch! plan. Your goal is to complete a minimum of thirty minutes of exercise five days a week at a moderate intensity.

I understand that changing your diet and beginning an exercise program at the same time can seem overwhelming. But I promise that if you follow my plan, it won't feel that way. In this chapter I'll help you find the time to walk by discovering hidden pockets in your schedule. I'll also help you get double-duty benefits by choosing one of four key mental/emotional payoffs every time you set out the door.

## the beauty of walking

The word *walk* comes from the Old English *wealcan,* which means "to roll." I love that, because when I walk, sometimes I feel like I'm gliding on wheels. Because my body inherently knows what to do (after all, I've been walking since around my first birthday), I can quickly get into a physical rhythm, which leaves my mind free to roam. Either I can connect with

## six more reasons to get moving

According to the Mayo Clinic, you can reap the following benefits from just thirty minutes of moderately intense exercise a day:

- **Lower blood pressure.** It's possible to lower your blood pressure by five to ten millimeters of mercury (mmHg), enough to cut back or even eliminate the need for blood-pressure medications.
- **Better cholesterol numbers.** Walking can reduce blood fats called triglycerides and increase your "good" HDL, the kind that helps keep your heart and arteries clear.
- **Improved blood-sugar control.** Exercise helps insulin work better. (Insulin is the hormone that keeps your blood sugar under control.)
- **Stronger bones.** Walking increases bone density and protects against the loss of bone tissue as you age.
- **Cancer prevention.** Walking helps reduce the risk of breast cancer by lowering body fat, a source of estrogen, which feeds breast-cancer cells. In a study published in the *Journal of the American Medical Association*, scientists tracked seventy-four thousand women for six years. Those between the ages of thirty-five and fifty who walked briskly for just one and a half to two hours per week had an 18 percent lower risk of being diagnosed with breast cancer later in life.
- **Better mental well-being.** Walking helps reduce stress, lessen feelings of depression and anxiety, improve sleep quality, and boost overall mood.

my surroundings and take in the sights, sounds, and smells, or I can tune them out and find the mental clarity that allows me to think through important issues, be creative (I came up with many of the recipes in this book while walking), or daydream. To me, walking feels like being in a "me time" bubble that I can use in whatever way I need to that day.

---

## another benefit to man's best friend

Dogs are a source of unconditional love, and studies show that pet ownership is associated with a lower risk of heart disease and fewer trips to the family doctor. Four-legged friends also help boost physical activity. Researchers found that dog owners exercised their pets an average of twice a day for twenty-four minutes each time—a total of five hours and thirty-six minutes a week—and that the pet owners were getting exercise at the same time. Pet owners also take their furry friends out on three long walks each week, adding another two hours and thirty-three minutes to the total. By comparison, those without a Fido or Spot who do exercise spend an average of just one hour and twenty minutes per week exercising, and nearly half (47 percent) say they get no exercise.

---

Some days, my walk allows me to think through important work-related or personal decisions. On other days, I conjure up my ultimate dream vacation or revisit a place I've been before that I fell in love with, like Hawaii or Paris. And sometimes when I walk, I mentally connect with my sister, who lives far away. Or I walk with my husband, and because there is no television or computer or pet to distract us, our walk really gives us time to bond. For all of these reasons, I not only look forward to walking but feel like it gives me something I don't want to live without.

While I'm walking, I'm aware that my heart and breathing rates rise, bringing me into "aerobic" exercise mode. And after I've walked, I feel and see the physical effects—a stronger body, better-quality sleep, and a more stable mood. When I'm out there, moving my feet and swinging my arms, walking doesn't mentally feel like work or a chore. In fact, just the opposite. Walking feels natural, and, well, for lack of a better word, it just feels *right!*

These are just some of the reasons that I enthusiastically recommend walking to my clients. Here are eight additional advantages:

- You don't need a gym membership.
- You can do it anywhere.
- You don't need any equipment, except for a sturdy pair of walking shoes; of course, if you find walking on a treadmill more convenient, that's a great option as well.
- You can do it year-round; as a New Yorker, I love the exhilaration I feel as I bundle up and head out to walk outdoors in the winter, with crunchy snow underfoot.
- You can walk alone, with your dog, or with a friend.
- There are no "rules" to walking.
- You already know how to do it.
- It can serve as a mental vacation from the chaos of everyday life.

## the four unique benefits of walking

Even if there were zero health benefits to walking and it didn't burn a single calorie, I'd still look forward to my daily walk because of what else it gives me. I can boil it down to four unique benefits. You can discover them, too! Try this assignment:

Take out a sheet of paper and make four columns. Then, write these four words, one at the top of each column:

Connect
Think
Dream
Bond

---

## what is metabolic syndrome?

Metabolic syndrome is a cluster of risk factors that raise the chances of developing heart disease, diabetes, and stroke. One-quarter of all U.S. adults qualify as having metabolic syndrome. To be diagnosed, you must have at least three of the following five risk factors:

- A large waistline—over thirty-five inches for women and over forty inches for men.
- High blood pressure—a level of 140/90 mmHg or higher. Normal is 120/80 mmHG.
- A high level of harmful triglycerides—normal is less than 150 mg/dL, and high is 200–499 mg/dL.
- Low "good" HDL cholesterol—60 mg/dL or higher is optimal, and low is less than 40 mg/dL for men or less than 50 mg/dL for women.
- High blood sugar—100 mg/dL (fasting level) is normal, and between 100 and 126 mg/dL is considered high.

---

**Connect** means connecting with your walking environment: feeling the air, taking in the sights and smells, and observing the people and nature around you. I live in New York City, so one day I may walk through the urban streets of Greenwich Village and another through Central Park, but every time that I'm in "connect" mode, I notice new things, even on streets I've walked down dozens of times, like the details of a building or the fashions in store windows. In the park, I spot gorgeous birds, and I love watching the resident squirrels chase each other through the lawn and up the trees. No two walks are ever the same, and I often feel like I'm on a minivacation, even when I'm in my own city. In this column, make a list of all the places you'd like to walk. Is there a park or nature center nearby or an area of town you've been meaning to explore? Be sure to include your own neighborhood.

**Think** means thinking through a personal or work-related situation that needs attention. Interruptions during the day, from phone calls and urgent e-mails to unexpected mishaps, like the kitchen sink clogging up, often prevent me from being able to focus on something that needs to be addressed. But during my walk, my blood gets pumping, and the flow of oxygen and nutrients to my brain, as well as the break from home or office distractions, gives me the clarity I need to reflect, consider my options, and determine how to proceed. In this column, list anything you feel you need to think through or focus on.

**Dream** means playful, creative time. The demands of everyday life probably leave you with little time to conjure up your fantasy vacation, consider new hobbies, or relish memories of your favorite past events. On one of my walks, I decided I wanted to finally learn to play guitar (something I had been thinking about for years, as I mentioned earlier), and when I got home, I immediately got online and signed up for a class, and I'm loving it. On other walks, I imagine what it would be like to live in some parts of the world I've visited, like Provence and Tokyo. As adults, our laundry list of daily responsibilities can leave us with little time to tap into our creativity the way we did as kids, but connecting to that part of ourselves is what helps us feel young, vibrant, and alive! In this column, write out all the things you wish you had more time to dream about.

**Bond** means bonding with the person you are walking with or the person you'd like to be walking with if he or she were in the same physical location. My sister and I are both big walkers, and we swear we sometimes have conversations with each other during our solo walks! Walking isn't my husband's favorite activity, but when we walk together, we have

24 25 26 27 28 29 30

I have sooo much energy. I feel like a well-oiled machine or an engine that has just been cleaned and is functioning more efficiently. My brain feels clear and clean. It's awesome!

MALEIKA, AGE 24

## these shoes were made for walking

If you head to a sporting-goods store, you'll probably find more shoes designed for walking than you can count on two hands. There's no "best" brand, and price isn't always the best indication of which shoe you should buy. When you try them on, search for the most comfortable fit for the length and width of your feet that accommodates your foot's arch type. Once you find a pair that feels comfy, make sure they give you enough cushioning and allow your feet flexibility and support at the same time. Walk around the store. The heel should fit snugly without slipping as you walk, and the entire shoe should feel pliable. Each time you take a step, your foot will "flex" as you roll from heel to toe. If a shoe is too stiff, your foot won't be able to bend properly, which will impede your walk. Finally, when you try on walking shoes, do so after you've been walking a while, when your feet are expanded, and wear the socks you'll be using when walking.

some of our best conversations, and by the time we get back home we're often holding hands (no small feat after thirteen years of marriage!). In this column, make a list of people you'd like to bond with. The list can include those you hope will become walking buddies—maybe a friend, neighbor, co-worker, or family member—and the people you want to bond with in your heart.

Each time you head out for your walk, set out to focus on one of these four benefits. Look over your lists, and zero in on what you feel best meets your needs that day. Investing in your walk in one of these four ways means you'll not only reap the benefits of exercise but also have a potent life-management tool that can help you meet both your emotional and social needs.

## finding the time to exercise

The chart on pages 244–45 is a tool I use with clients who say they don't have time to shop, cook, or exercise. This week, fill in exactly how you spend every thirty-minute block of time. Be as specific as possible, and if you do more than one task in a thirty-minute period, such as spending fifteen minutes on the phone and fifteen checking e-mails, be sure to note this. I know that filling out a time chart can feel like yet another task to complete in your already overflowing schedule, but it's actually the only way to really know how you're spending your days.

In many ways, a time chart is a lot like a food diary. Most of my clients really believe they're eating lots of fruits and veggies, but when they complete a food journal and add it up, they typically find that what seemed like five servings a day turned out to be two. When I filled out my time chart, I found that I was sleeping a lot less than I thought and wasting more time than I realized! Instead of viewing this as a homework assignment, think of it as a journey of self-exploration. You might be surprised at what you'll learn.

Once you've filled out the time chart, analyze your results. No doubt you will find spots in your day that include "nonessential" activities, such as web surfing or watching a show that doesn't exactly qualify as "must-see TV." These are the slots to fill in with a walk. Or, instead of talking on the phone with a neighbor or friend, invite him or her to walk with you.

Here's some great news for busy people: research shows that completing three ten-minute sessions or two fifteen-minute blocks is just as beneficial as one thirty-minute walk. I have no doubt that you can carve out small blocks of time to walk! Think through your daily schedule, and use the following chart to note those times, on at least five days, when you'll commit to walking for a daily total of thirty minutes:

Monday Walk Time(s):
Tuesday Walk Time(s):
Wednesday Walk Time(s):
Thursday Walk Time(s):
Friday Walk Time(s):
Saturday Walk Time(s):
Sunday Walk Time(s):

**cinch!**

| TIME | MON | TUE | WED | THU | FRI | SAT | SUN |
|---|---|---|---|---|---|---|---|
| 5:00–5:30 A.M. | | | | | | | |
| 5:30–6:00 A.M. | | | | | | | |
| 6:00–6:30 A.M. | | | | | | | |
| 6:30–7:00 A.M. | | | | | | | |
| 7:00–7:30 A.M. | | | | | | | |
| 7:30–8:00 A.M. | | | | | | | |
| 8:00–8:30 A.M. | | | | | | | |
| 8:30–9:00 A.M. | | | | | | | |
| 9:00–9:30 A.M. | | | | | | | |
| 9:30–10:00 A.M. | | | | | | | |
| 10:00–10:30 A.M. | | | | | | | |
| 10:30–11:00 A.M. | | | | | | | |
| 11:00–11:30 A.M. | | | | | | | |
| 11:30–12:00 P.M. | | | | | | | |
| 12:00–12:30 P.M. | | | | | | | |
| 12:30–1:00 P.M. | | | | | | | |
| 1:00–1:30 P.M. | | | | | | | |
| 1:30–2:00 P.M. | | | | | | | |
| 2:00–2:30 P.M. | | | | | | | |
| 2:30–3:00 P.M. | | | | | | | |
| 3:00–3:30 P.M. | | | | | | | |
| 3:30–4:00 P.M. | | | | | | | |
| 4:00–4:30 P.M. | | | | | | | |
| 4:30–5:00 P.M. | | | | | | | |

| TIME | MON | TUE | WED | THU | FRI | SAT | SUN |
|---|---|---|---|---|---|---|---|
| 5:00–5:30 P.M. | | | | | | | |
| 5:30–6:00 P.M. | | | | | | | |
| 6:00–6:30 P.M. | | | | | | | |
| 6:30–7:00 P.M. | | | | | | | |
| 7:00–7:30 P.M. | | | | | | | |
| 7:30–8:00 P.M. | | | | | | | |
| 8:00–8:30 P.M. | | | | | | | |
| 8:30–9:00 P.M. | | | | | | | |
| 9:00–9:30 P.M. | | | | | | | |
| 9:30–10:00 P.M. | | | | | | | |
| 10:00–10:30 P.M. | | | | | | | |
| 10:30–11:00 P.M. | | | | | | | |
| 11:00–11:30 P.M. | | | | | | | |
| 11:30–12:00 A.M. | | | | | | | |
| 12:00–12:30 A.M. | | | | | | | |
| 12:30–1:00 A.M. | | | | | | | |
| 1:00–1:30 A.M. | | | | | | | |
| 1:30–2:00 A.M. | | | | | | | |
| 2:00–2:30 A.M. | | | | | | | |
| 2:30–3:00 A.M. | | | | | | | |
| 3:00–3:30 A.M. | | | | | | | |
| 3:30–4:00 A.M. | | | | | | | |
| 4:00–4:30 A.M. | | | | | | | |
| 4:30–5:00 A.M. | | | | | | | |

Now that you have identified when you can walk and for how long and you've made a commitment to do it, let's talk about how fast. To reap all the benefits I've discussed, you need to engage in moderate exercise—in other words, activities significantly more challenging than your daily routine.

To gauge intensity, think of a scale from zero to ten. Zero is sitting, reading this book. Ten is pushing yourself to the max—maybe jumping rope or sprinting. If you've been inactive, start out at a pace that feels like a six to an eight on that scale. You'll find that the more you walk and the more your body adjusts, even within days, the walking speed that used to register as an eight will slide down to a six.

When you walk as transportation, like walking to the mailbox or library in your neighborhood, your average speed is probably about three miles per hour. In other words, in thirty minutes you cover about a mile and a half. That's not quite fast enough to count as moderate, so you need a concrete way to measure your intensity.

Distance-per-thirty-minutes is one good way. As you begin walking, track your distance. Four miles per hour, or a distance of one mile every fifteen minutes, is considered a moderate pace. If you enjoy using a pedometer, a rate of at least one hundred steps per minute counts as moderately intense exercise, according to a study published in the *American Journal of Preventive Medicine*. So during a thirty-minute walking session, aim for three thousand steps. If that seems like too quick a pace at first, work your way up gradually. You'll be amazed at how quickly your body will adjust.

Should you work your way up to running? I don't think so. Sometimes, when a runner whizzes by me, I contemplate breaking into a jog, but I stop myself for a few reasons. As a former runner, I know that walking is much less stressful on my body. With walking, one foot remains on the ground, whereas with running, both feet are "in the air" with each step. The gravity-induced impact or "pounding" on your frame from running may lead to an increased risk of injury and arthritic joints. Also, research shows that walking is just as effective for health and weight control when the same distance is covered. A Duke University study found

## the afterburn myth

After a great walk, I have to remind myself that I didn't just run a marathon. Like many of my clients, I can be susceptible to the "But I worked out today" mindset that can lead to extra nibbling. The truth is, the number of calories you burn while exercising is mostly tied to your weight. (The less you weigh, the less you burn.) Even during a moderately intense hour of cardio, I burn only about 350 calories—the equivalent of a large soy latte and a banana. Though it's true that you do burn more calories per hour after your workout ends, it's not enough to sanction a splurge.

One study found that premenopausal women who did forty minutes of cardio at 80 percent of their maximum heart rate (think eight on an intensity scale of zero to ten) burned more calories for up to sixty-seven hours, but the "afterburn" amounted to just 15 percent—a total of fifty additional calories. Bottom line: think of your walks as a way to burn extra fat, not a way to earn extra calories. Fortunately, researchers at the University of Exeter have found that walking, even just fifteen minutes a day, can reduce your cravings for sweets!

that over eight months, thirty-minute-a-day walkers who logged about twelve miles per week lost 1 percent of their body weight, 2 percent of their body fat, and 1.6 percent of their waist circumference; those who jogged twelve miles per week lost 1 percent of their body weight, 2.6 percent of their body fat, and 1.4 percent of their waist circumference. The results were virtually identical!

# get inspired today!

If you're still struggling with the idea of lacing up your shoes, try this exercise, which I do with my clients. Take out a sheet of paper, and list the pros and cons of adding walking to your schedule. What will you get from walking, and what will you give up? As you look over your responses, rank them in importance to you right now. For example, under pros you may have listed weight loss, better sleep, and stress relief, but under cons you might have included that you'd rather spend the little free time you have doing something else such as reading. Of everything you listed, how would you rank their significance to you right now? Your answer will give you an important insight into how ready you are.

List any preparation you think you need to do before you can begin your walking routine. For example, in addition to filling out the time chart and planning when you'll walk, do you need to buy shoes or socks, get a new leash for your dog, or find a walking buddy? Thinking through what you'll need to do to prepare for walking can help you feel more ready to move ahead.

On a scale from zero to ten, how confident do you feel about your ability to begin and maintain a walking program? Zero would be no confidence, and ten fully confident. If your answer isn't ten, what would help you feel more self-assured? A lot of my clients gain confidence when they begin to rack more steps per minute or a greater distance per hour.

Cinch! isn't about eating right and being active because you're supposed to. It's about learning how to take care of yourself in ways that make you feel amazing inside and out. By the end of your thirty-day journey, walking will be an activity you look forward to, with major payoffs. You'll shrink your fat cells, improve your health from head to toe, and enjoy a near-daily dose of priceless "you" time. Get ready to fall in love with walking!

# 10

24 25 26 27 28 29 30 31 32 33

# just in case you asked . . .

I n other chapters I have included all the information necessary for following Cinch!, but there are some queries I frequently hear from clients that just didn't fall neatly into a particular chapter. I've included them here. If you still have questions after reading this chapter, please visit www.cinchyourself.com. There you'll find more tips, information, and resources, and you can message me directly.

## weight-loss questions

*Why does my weight fluctuate from day to day?*

Your weight as a number is fickle. When you step on the scale, it simultaneously measures the weight of seven things: (1) muscle; (2) bone; (3) organs, like your lungs, heart, and liver; (4) fluids, including blood;

(5) body fat; (6) the waste inside your digestive tract that you haven't yet eliminated; and (7) glycogen, the form of carbohydrate you sock away in your liver and muscles, which serves as a backup fuel or energy piggy bank. Any change on the scale is due to a loss or gain of one or more of these substances, and some—especially your fluids, waste, and glycogen—fluctuate more readily than others.

For example, two cups of water weighs one pound, so a shift in water has an immediate impact on your overall weight. Constipation also can cause you to weigh more until your body releases the waste it's hanging on to. And if you eat slightly more or less carbohydrate from one day to the next, your glycogen stores fluctuate as well. For these reasons, it's actually normal for your weight to ebb and flow, so if you see it slightly increase from one day to the next, don't panic, and remember these three facts:

1. You can be losing body fat and retaining water at the same time, which means your weight on the scale can increase while you're slimming down.

2. To gain just one pound of actual body fat, you'd have to eat 3,500 more calories than you burn, which is a lot of extra eating (think 500 excess calories every day for seven days straight—500 is the amount in three handfuls of potato chips, a slice of pecan pie, or a cup of premium ice cream). If your weight on the scale increases by one pound and you haven't consumed an excess 3,500 calories, you haven't actually gained a pound of body fat.

3. Instead of watching how your weight changes from day to day, it's more important to focus on how your body size changes over time. Your clothes should fit a little looser each week. And remember, you may be "shrinking" and whittling away body fat even if the number on the scale hasn't budged.

*Why are my husband and my friend losing weight faster than I am?*
There are several reasons that two people following the same plan lose weight at different rates. As I mentioned earlier, when you step on a scale, you're not just measuring a change in body fat. The bigger and taller a

# how to build in a splurge

As much as I love and believe in this plan, sometimes even I have to get my french-fry fix! That's why I included this section about how to stick to the Cinch! strategy most of the time and build in some strategic splurges. Here's how it works:

1.   Zero in on your target. Figure out what you really, really want: What's going to do it for you? Are you craving a specific food like chips, potatoes, or red meat, or a texture or flavor as well—salty or sweet, hot or chilled, creamy or crispy?

2.   Get your fix—but use a strategy. Once you know precisely what you want, find a way to get just the right amount of a high-quality version and think about how to incorporate it into a meal by eating your can't-live-without food in place of some of the puzzle pieces.

For example, potatoes are very starchy, so french fries or potato chips, which are cooked in oil, would be closest to the whole-grain and plant-based-fat puzzle pieces. A good strategy would be to have a serving of chips or fries with grilled veggies and shrimp. If you're craving red meat, maybe you have a burger or steak in place of your usual salmon, along with the rest of the puzzle pieces, like a small piece of tenderloin with wild rice and a garden salad with balsamic vinegar and extra-virgin olive oil.

Baked goods like cookies are closest to the whole-grain and plant-based-fat pieces, so a savvy approach would be to buy one freshly baked cookie, brownie, or cupcake from a really great bakery (instead of a bag or box) and enjoy it after eating your lean protein and veggies. If ice cream's your thing, swap out a scoop of premium ice cream for the lean-protein, whole-grain, and plant-based-fat puzzle pieces. For example, enjoy a half cup of your favorite flavor ice cream topped with fresh or grilled in-season fruit as a snack meal, or eat some grilled veggie kabobs with a small scoop of ice cream for dessert.

Most of your splurge foods probably won't contain whole grains, lean protein, or plant-based fat, but they will contain carbohydrates, protein, and fat, which are components of what those puzzle pieces give to your body. To avoid doubling up, use this cheat sheet to sub in for your splurge:

- Potatoes, refined flour, and sugar provide carbohydrates, so they are closest to the whole-grain puzzle piece.
- Red meat provides protein, so it is closest to the lean-protein puzzle piece.

- Ice cream provides carbohydrate, some protein, and fat, so it is closest to the lean-protein, whole-grain, and plant-based-fat puzzle pieces.
- Pizza provides carbohydrates, protein, and fat, so it is closest to the whole-grain, lean-protein, and plant-based-fat puzzle pieces. It probably doesn't provide enough veggies to count as the produce piece as well, so pairing a slice of pizza with a salad dressed with balsamic vinegar would be a smart splurge strategy.

As far as how often to splurge, I recommend no more than once a week, preferably after thirty solid days of following the Cinch! strategy. A Friday-night dinner or Sunday-brunch splurge and consistent Cinch! strategy the rest of the week should allow you to continue to lose weight and maintain your results, but I do think that listening to your body is also key. You know your body better than anyone, so if you pay attention in terms of how a splurge impacts your energy, digestion, return of hunger, and so forth, I think you will quickly see the best way to have your cake and eat it too!

Personally, building a splurge into the puzzle principle feels best, because it's satisfying but I can still maintain my weight and it doesn't completely throw off my body. If you really go all out (burger and fries with dessert), it may take two or three days to get back to normal in terms of hunger, appetite, digestion, and even how your clothes fit.

In all my years of working with clients, I've had so many tell me that they were all geared up for a big splurge and afterward felt really disappointed because either the food wasn't all that great or worth it, or they felt so awful by the end of the meal (sluggish, sleepy, bloated) that it wasn't an enjoyable experience. But a more balanced splurge, like ordering grilled fish and veggies at a restaurant and replacing the whole-grain and plant-based-fat puzzle pieces for a dessert feels much closer to the "Goldilocks" result—satisfying but still energizing.

Finally, if you find yourself dreaming about cheesecake or a T-bone steak, check in with your emotions. You may find that your craving is less about the food and more about how you're feeling. If that's the case, revisit the exercises in chapter 8 to sort out your thoughts and feelings. If what you really need is comfort or an escape, you may just find that food isn't the best panacea.

person is, the more fluid, waste, and glycogen he or she carries, which means that person has more of these to lose. In addition, the bigger and taller a person is, the more calories he or she burns, both at rest and during exercise, so it's easier for a bigger person to create the 3,500-calorie deficit needed to lose one pound of true body fat. For example, a 200-pound man burns 200 more calories per hour than a 145-pound woman when both walk at a speed of five miles per hour. So, although this may seem completely unfair, try to put your smaller but steady weight loss in perspective and celebrate *your* success.

### What do I do if I fall off track?

For whatever reason, from a really bad day to a major celebration, if you find yourself off track at some point, follow this five-step fix:

1. Do a quick reality check. As bloated and heavy as you may feel, remember that it takes an excess 3,500 calories to gain just one pound of true body fat. Two glasses of wine and tiramisu add up to about 750; a whole basket of tortilla chips with guacamole and a margarita is 850. I'm definitely not encouraging you to stray from this plan, because I want you to see results and look and feel your best, but keep in mind that a onetime splurge may not derail your weight as much as you think. Bottom line: overeating by a few hundred calories every day, week after week, is a lot more damaging than a single episode of indulging.

2. Be sure to get back on track with your water intake—a total of two and a half liters (eight to ten cups) per day. Water will help flush out any excess sodium you're hanging on to, which could be causing water retention. Water is attracted to sodium like a magnet; that's

> Making time to cook every night was definitely a change I had to make, so I found little things that sped up the process. I make two dinners and eat the second for lunch the next day. Also before I start cooking all my meals, I get out every single ingredient I'll need. I've found this really speeds up the process.
>
> AMY, AGE 28

why you hang on to more when you eat saltier meals. And two cups of water weighs one pound. So drinking yourself back into sodium balance can help you see a faster downward blip on your bathroom scale.

3. Get back to Fast Forward meals. You may be tempted to cut back even more, but starving yourself after a slight deviation can backfire because it can slow down your metabolism, causing you to hang on to any fat you may have stored. Just resume your regular plan, and be as consistent as possible with the timing of your meals to get your digestive system and metabolism back on track. If you really went full tilt (like a day of bingeing), just repeat the Fast Forward, but three days instead of five should be enough to undo the damage.

4. Choose fiber-rich foods. Bulking up on fiber will help get things moving through your system, so to speak. That's key, since an unusually heavy day of eating can lead to short-term constipation. Also, fiber is filling, but fiber itself doesn't contribute calories to your diet, since it doesn't get digested or absorbed. Some of the best sources of fiber are pears, apples, berries, beans, whole-wheat pasta, barley, artichokes, and broccoli. Look for Cinch! meals that include these foods.

5. Boost your activity level. Adding an extra fifteen minutes to your walk can help you pay off the calorie debt you've racked up. Think of it as working extra hours to pay off holiday bills. Even parking your car farther away and walking briskly an extra fifteen minutes a day burns an additional 85 calories. And psychologically, sweating a little more can help you feel like you've put your calorie checkbook back into balance.

> My friends claim that it was impossible to feel full after my salad but I did.
>
> RENEE, AGE 45

### How can I reduce bloating?

Bloating is typically caused by a buildup of gas inside your digestive tract. The gas can be swallowed—from carbonated drinks, skipping meals (air contains gases), eating too quickly, or chewing gum (which I don't recommend for this reason and because gum contains either added sugar or sugar substitutes, and often artificial additives). All of these cause extra air to be swallowed and trapped in your belly. Gas can build up when bacteria attack undigested portions of food, and it can be caused by lactose intolerance in people who lack the enzyme needed to digest lactose, the natural sugar in milk. Sometimes gas can be brought on by foods that irritate the delicate lining of the GI tract, like spicy peppers or acidic foods such as coffee and tomato sauce. Stress, lack of sleep, hormonal changes, and an erratic eating pattern also can be culprits. A food diary in which you track your habits and symptoms can be the best way to identify your personal triggers, but if you feel chronically bloated, and if making changes such as eating slower and avoiding dairy doesn't help, see your doctor.

*I have considered getting liposuction. What are your feelings about plastic surgery?*

I think plastic surgery of any kind is a very personal decision, but in my experience, you can achieve safer, better-than-liposuction results by following this plan. A recent survey found that 83 percent of women want liposuction, and 40 percent would have it if it were free. Each year, nearly 350,000 men and women undergo this procedure; that's equal to the entire population of Tampa, Florida. According to the FDA, deaths associated with liposuction are higher than fatalities from car crashes. The fatality rate could be as high as between twenty and one hundred per hundred thousand procedures, according to the FDA. The death rate from car accidents is only sixteen per hundred thousand crashes. Liposuction also is expensive; costs can vary, but I've often seen fees of approximately thirty-five hundred dollars for one body part, sixty-eight hundred dollars for two body parts, and ninety-seven hundred dollars for five body parts.

Cinch! has done wonders for me. I feel great and look great. LISSELY, AGE 29

For all that, liposuction is actually less effective than a diet-and-exercise approach. The maximum amount of fat that can be removed safely in liposuction is six to eight pounds. Removing more in a single procedure increases the risk of serious complications. And you won't see the ultimate results until one to three months postsurgery. In terms of long-term complications, some studies have shown that surgical removal of subcutaneous fat (under the skin) may contribute to an increase in visceral fat (deep, internal fat around major organs), the most dangerous type of fat to have on your body. And the side effects of lipo can include scars; saggy, lumpy skin; and weight regain in all the wrong places. If a woman has liposuction on her hips, outer thighs, and belly and then gains ten pounds, she'll gain it in areas where fat cells haven't been removed, such as her face, neck, back, and legs. If she ultimately gains a lot of weight, it can come back in the areas where lipo was performed.

Finding a healthful, balanced way of eating that you can maintain forever is a much safer, faster, far less expensive, all-natural alternative to cosmetic surgery. By the time you finish this thirty-day plan, the "L" word will be purged from your vocabulary!

*How do I help my husband lose weight?*

Most people gain weight after marriage—an average of fifteen to thirty pounds over five years, according to a recent study, but you can buck the trend. When I met my husband, Jack, he was fifty-plus pounds overweight and had a long list of horrific eating habits. Fast forward twelve years: I'm the same size, and he has shed seven inches from his belly—but I never once forced, tricked, bribed, or coerced him into eating healthier. Here are my 100 percent nag-free tips for helping your hubby "healthy up":

- Ban the "f" word (*fat*). Don't bring up the size of his belly. Making his weight the issue can put him on the defensive, make him feel resentful, result in spiteful unhealthy eating, and build a wall between the two of you. Instead, focus on what will motivate him today, like having more energy or looking younger, and make it a team effort instead of singling him out.

- Offer; don't preach. Research shows that unhealthy habits are so-cially contagious, but healthy ones rub off, too. The best results happen organically, in a positive environment. Offer him some of your Berry Almond French Toast at breakfast, or water instead of cola, but don't push. If the words "You shouldn't be eating that" or "You don't eat enough vegetables" come out of your mouth, you'll likely wind up in an ugly behavioral tug-of-war.

- Put yourself in his shoes. The foundation of any change is readiness. Think back to how you felt before you began this plan. If someone had tried to push you before you were ready, you probably would have pushed back. If he's not quite there yet, be patient. I know it's tough to see pepperoni grease dripping down the chin of the guy you love, but ultimately, he has to want to make the change.

## personal health questions

*Is this plan appropriate for someone following a low-sodium diet?*

Yes. The maximum daily sodium recommendation is 1,500 to 2,300 mg, yet the average person consumes 3,400 mg or more per day. Seventy percent of that comes from processed foods, which this plan greatly minimizes. You'll be building the majority of your meals from whole foods—like veggies, whole grains, and lean proteins—instead of stuff that comes in cans or boxes. But when you do buy packaged foods, remember these tips:

- Check out the number of milligrams of sodium. It's not realistic to add up every milligram all day long, but comparing the amount in a given food to the daily limit of 1,500 to 2,300 is a great way to gauge how much you're "spending" and contrast similar foods, like two different kinds of bread. Some foods may surprise you. For example, salted almonds have only 110 mg of sodium per quarter-cup serving. That's because sodium isn't processed into the food;

it's just a light seasoning on the outside. By contrast, a cinnamon scone—a snack you wouldn't consider "salty"—contains 510 mg of sodium. Generally, the more processed a food is, the higher the amount of sodium. For example, a single serving of frozen pizza can pack over 1,800 mg!

- Keep in mind that the words *reduced sodium* on a food label don't mean low sodium. "Reduced sodium" means the sodium was reduced by at least 25 percent from its original amount.
- Be sure to check every packaged food. You may find high amounts of sodium in some foods that don't taste salty, such as some types of cereal.

Finally, one of the best ways to keep sodium under control is to eat more potassium, unless you've been told to avoid it by your doctor. Potassium acts as a natural diuretic, so it sweeps excess sodium and water out of your body. Potassium-rich foods include bananas, spinach, yogurt, and avocados, which are all built into the meals in chapter 4.

*Do you recommend taking supplements?*

I take probiotics, vegetarian omega-3s, and vegetarian vitamin D, and recommend these three supplements to most of my clients, but I don't believe that supplement recommendations should be one-size-fits-all. The types and amounts of supplements you use should be based on filling a gap that can't be filled by changing your diet. That said, it's difficult for most people (including me) to get enough probiotics, omega-3 fatty acids, and vitamin D through food alone. For years I've been taking a daily capsule of Nature's Way Primadophilus Bifidus. Each contains 5 billion CFUs, or colony-forming units, which are a measure of how many bacteria are able to divide and form colonies; this indicates that the probiotics are alive and healthy. Five billion is the amount I and many other health professionals recommend for reaping the benefits of these "good bugs," which include improving digestion, boosting immunity, and, as I mention on page 48, possibly playing a role in weight management. Because

I eat a plant-based diet, I take a vegan form of vitamin D made by VegLife, but many of my clients take an animal-based form of D, which is typically derived from seafood but sometimes from sheep's wool, hides, or other animal parts.

As I mention on page 263, due to the risks of mercury and other contamination, you should limit seafood to no more than twelve ounces of seafood per week, if you eat it at all. But even if you love salmon and shrimp, it's difficult to reach the recommended 1,000 mg per day (combined) of the essential DHA and EPA omega-3 fatty acids. I don't eat seafood, so I get my omega-3s from a vegetarian supplement called NutraVege, made by Ascenta, that contains DHA from algae (which is where fish get their DHA). It's also formulated with echium oil, which is derived from a flowering plant that contains a type of fat that gets converted into EPA in the body. In addition to NutraVege, Ascenta makes several fish-oil products from sustainably sourced sardines and anchovies. I visited their facilities in Nova Scotia and was blown away by the purity and quality. What truly sets this brand apart is a unique program they created called Pure Check. Pure Check means that every bottle they produce is tested by an independent third-party lab to verify that the amount of omega-3s listed is accurate, the oil hasn't degraded, and it's free from heavy-metal contamination, including mercury, lead, dioxins, PCBs, and others. Only after the results are reviewed and verified are the bottles shipped to markets, and each bottle contains a lot number that allows you to view the Pure Check report for your specific batch online. Every supplement manufacturer should operate this way. Because dietary supplements aren't regulated in the same way prescription drugs are, there is no guarantee that any supplement you buy is safe, effective, contains what the label states, and is free from contaminants. Ascenta is the only brand I've ever seen that voluntarily verifies

> 24 25 26 27 28 29 30
>
> Building a Cinch! meal with the components is almost like shopping for a new wardrobe—you pick out your main staples that can be mixed and matched—it is all about pairing things properly and throwing on the right accessories!
>
> JESSICA, AGE 32

their products. I was so impressed with this company that I began to develop recipes with their products, but I usually take my all-natural citrus-flavored NutraVege right from the spoon. To learn more about Ascenta and Pure Check visit www.ascentahealth.com. To decide which supplements may be right for you and how much and how often you should take them, talk to your doctor or your personal dietitian.

*I want to start this plan, but I just started dating someone. What should I do?*

If you're ready to start, don't hesitate. I think it's important not to hide your true food personality at the start of a relationship. I've counseled many couples who end up fighting about food constantly because one disguised his or her true food colors from the partner early on.

For example, some women will go "guy style"—drinking beer, eating chicken wings, and ordering steak—because they think that's what a guy wants, even when it's the opposite of how they really want to eat. Once a couple settles into a comfort zone, the "food faker" will eventually be revealed, so I say: be up front at the start. Truly understanding and accepting how the other eats is a big part of a relationship, because couples spend more time eating than doing just about anything else together. If a guy knows right away that this is your way of eating, he can either accept it (and not ask you to split a pint of Häagen-Dazs or a pizza while watching TV) or decide that it's a deal breaker. You don't need to spill every detail of your eating habits on the first date, but don't stray too far from what's truly "you."

## grocery-related questions

*Why is there no salt in any of the meals?*

As I mention on page 72, salt has become a major nutritional villain. In the United States, the maximum daily sodium recommendation is 1,500 to 2,300 mg, but according to a recent study, the average American consumes about 3,400 mg per day, and other estimates peg our daily intake at a much higher 10,000 mg.

Earlier in my career, I worked in cardiac rehab. For people with heart disease, restricting salt and sodium is very important, because too much can raise blood pressure and worsen heart disease. But today, most of my private-practice clients are athletes and relatively healthy adults who are trying to lose weight; so when it comes to sodium, I'm often asked, "Do I really need to pay attention to this?" The answer is definitely yes. Salty foods tend to increase thirst, and you may be tempted to quench that thirst with beverages packed with calories. Also, salt enhances the taste of foods and therefore may encourage overeating, and finally, there is some animal research to show that a high-sodium diet may affect the activity of fat cells, making them larger. In addition, fluid is attracted to sodium like a magnet, so when you take in too much, you retain more water, which means bloating and puffiness. For these reasons I decided not to include salt as a SASS.

As a health professional, I want you to reach your weight goal in a way that will also keep you well and prevent the chronic diseases that may run in your family. Reducing sodium is an important preventative medicine strategy, and fortunately it's relatively easy to do. About 70 percent of the sodium in the American diet is from processed foods. By eating more fresh, whole foods, which you are with this plan, you're automatically slashing your sodium intake. For example, ½ cup cooked whole oats with 2 tablespoons walnut butter; 1 cup fresh strawberries, seasoned with cinnamon, nutmeg, and cloves; and 1 cup of organic soy milk contains a mere 132 mg of sodium. And one of my favorite salad concoctions—1 cup organic mixed greens; ¼ cup each grape tomatoes, red onion, shredded carrots, and sliced mushrooms; ½ cup cooked, chilled broad beans; ½ cup cooked, chilled quinoa; ¼ ripe Hass avocado; 2 tablespoons balsamic vinegar; a squeeze of fresh lemon; and ¼ teaspoon freshly ground pepper—packs less than 300 mg. By comparison, a low-calorie frozen dinner contains about 700 mg and a 6-inch turkey sub on wheat from Subway packs over 900 mg. The only exception to limiting salt in healthy adults is for athletes or people who engage in activities that cause them to lose a lot of sodium in their sweat. But when that's the case, processed foods aren't the best way to replace sodium. Just one level teaspoon of sea salt packs 2,360 mg of sodium. If your meals provide 300 mg of sodium on average, your four meals a day will add up to 1,200 mg, but your sodium intake may be more or less depending on the ingredients you choose. A half cup of nonfat cottage cheese can have 380 mg of sodium alone and a half cup of canned black beans can pack 460 mg (although rinsing them can wash away 40 percent of that), while 1 serving of tofu has 0 mg of sodium.

If you feel that you are losing a lot of sodium in sweat and you think you might need to include some salt in your meals to replace your losses, try to limit your intake to no more than one level teaspoon per day of all-natural salt, such as sea salt or an exotic natural variety such as Himalayan Pink (from ancient sea salt deposits in the Himalayan Mountains), Rose Salt (from the Andes Mountains of Bolivia), Hawaiian Black Lava Salt, or Fleur de Sel (considered to be the finest of all sea salts).

*Should I worry about mercury in seafood?*

Yes. Mercury is a serious issue, and it affects all of us. A study in over six thousand American women found that blood levels of mercury are accumulating, and high levels in adults have been linked to heart disease and Alzheimer's. The report, from the Centers for Disease Control and Prevention, found that mercury was detected in the blood of 30 percent of women aged eighteen to forty-nine in the 2005–2006 *National Health and Nutrition Report,* compared with just 2 percent of women in the 1999–2000 report—an astonishing increase. On the other hand, seafood is high in protein, low in saturated fat, and a rich source of omega-3 fatty acids, which are important for heart health and baby brain development and possibly valuable for fighting mental decline, depression, stroke, and inflammation. If you're a seafood lover, here's what you need to know to keep yourself safe:

- The five most commonly eaten fish that are low in mercury are shrimp, canned chunk light tuna, salmon, pollack, and catfish. Eat these varieties more frequently than other types of seafood. The Environmental Defense Fund's seafood selector, online at www.edf.org/page.cfm?tagID=1521, can help you choose the seafood that is lowest in mercury and best for the environment.
- Eat no more than twelve ounces of seafood per week.
- Avoid seafood known to be high in mercury, which includes shark, swordfish, king mackerel, and tilefish. (I have not included these four types in any of my meals.)
- Check your exposure. Safe levels of mercury also have to do with your body weight. You can find calculators online that allow you to plug in your weight and seafood intake and show you how much mercury you're taking in. Visit www.gotmercury.org and www.nrdc.org/health/effects/mercury/calculator/start.asp. And to learn about sustainable seafood, visit www.seafoodwatch.org.

*When I go to the market, there's a wall of bread. How do I know which one to buy?*

The bread aisle does seem to be expanding! There used to be your basic white or wheat, and now there are rows of choices, and picking the healthiest one can be tricky. Here's what you need to know:

- Check the ingredient list first. Select breads made only with ingredients you'd use to make bread in your kitchen: whole grains, water, yeast, and salt. Yes, breads without added preservatives will go moldy quickly, so if you buy a fresh loaf, and you don't think you'll use it within a few days, store it in the freezer. You can quickly thaw out a few slices on the countertop or toast it. Some preservative-free breads are sold in the freezer section.
- Try out not just whole-wheat breads but also breads made from other whole grains or from multiple grains like oats, rye, and barley. You'll find some made with over a dozen different varieties.

Just remember that "twelve-grain bread" isn't any healthier than one-grain bread unless the label says it's "100 percent whole grain."

*Why can't I use 2 percent milk?*

Two percent sounds lean, and it does contain less fat than whole milk, but that percentage represents the *weight* of the milk that's fat, not the percentage of calories from fat. If 2 percent milk wasn't homogenized (mixed together), you'd see that more than one-third of each glass is pure fat—mostly saturated fat, the solid kind that clogs arteries and increases the risk of heart disease. The percentage of calories from fat in 2 percent milk is actually 35 percent. According to the *Dietary Guidelines for Americans,* everyone two years old and older should be drinking 1 percent or skim milk, both of which contain the same amount of protein and calcium as 2 percent.

*I've heard that grilling is unhealthy. Why did you include grilled options?*

It's true that cooking meat to high temperatures can trigger the formation of three known cancer-causing substances, but I don't think you need to give your grill the pink slip just yet. Here's why:

- There is safety in your SASS. Marinating even briefly before grilling has been shown to decrease the formation of these risky substances by over 90 percent. Also, a Kansas State University study found that adding rosemary to the surface of meats before grilling caused the levels of these substances to plummet by 30 to 100 percent.
- Some of the risky substances are formed when fat drips onto coals or stones, creating smoke and flare-ups that settle back onto your food. Because you'll be grilling only ultralean poultry or seafood, there will be few, if any, drippings. You also can keep flare-ups under control by spreading aluminum foil on the grill, perforated with small holes to allow any fat to drain through. It also helps to precut your meat so it doesn't need to spend as much time on the

grill. Flipping the meat frequently also speeds cooking time and helps prevent these substances from forming.

* Your plate offers protection. To offset the effects of grilling, the American Institute for Cancer Research recommends filling about one-third of your plate or less with grilled meat or seafood and at least two-thirds with plant-based foods. That's because the antioxidants and natural substances found in veggies and whole grains are cancer protective. And research shows that plant-based foods help stimulate enzymes that deactivate cancer-causing compounds. On this plan, the proportion of your plate will always follow this guideline.

*Why do you emphasize buying food produced locally?*

For one thing, locally grown produce is allowed to reach its peak maturity, whereas fruits and veggies grown far away are often picked early and artificially ripened to extend their shelf life. This means local produce develops higher levels of the natural antioxidants that heighten their smell and taste. If you've ever picked a berry from the bush and popped it into your mouth or plucked a tomato from your garden minutes before adding it to your salad, you've experienced this difference in aroma and taste intensity.

Eating in-season produce soon after harvest maximizes enjoyment and can lead to more fruits and veggies ending up on your plate and in your body rather than rotting in the crisper. If you can, get out to a pick-your-own farm. When you see how and where food is grown, get to meet the people who grow it, and have the chance to harvest it yourself, you can't help but feel the connection between how plants are nourished and how they nourish you. And when you visit farms, you truly understand why it's not natural to eat watermelon in the middle of winter!

*Do you recommend reduced-fat products?*

No. Aside from dairy products, which provide the same amount of protein and nutrients without the saturated fat, I'm not a big fan of reduced-fat foods. For example, reduced-fat peanut butter has about the same number of calories per serving as regular peanut butter and usually more sugar. (There are plenty of brands of natural nut butters that have no sugar at all; these are the ones I recommend.) It's hard for manufacturers to take out the fat, so they have to add sugar or carbs to displace the fat content. To achieve a lower fat level per serving, they have to add something to displace the fat. Compare the ingredients, and you'll spot the extras. Plus, the fat in peanut butter is heart-healthy, monounsaturated fat, aka MUFA, so you don't want less fat per serving. When buying packaged foods, stick with all-natural versions, including regular nut butters such as peanut, almond, cashew, walnut, and sunflower.

*Is any type of ground turkey okay on this plan?*

No. You need to look at the percentage that is lean. Choose at least 93 percent lean, and go even higher if you can find it: 99 percent lean ground turkey has 40 percent fewer calories per serving than 93 percent lean ground turkey. You can also find the leanest turkey or chicken breast you can buy and ask for it to be ground at the meat counter.

*Can I use veggie wraps in place of pita or corn tortillas?*

No. Veggie wraps, like spinach or sun-dried tomato wraps, don't count toward your daily veggie intake. In fact, many brands are made with white flour, and the veggie is included only as a scant seasoning ingredient that makes up less than 2 percent of the wrap. Instead, stick with 100 percent whole-grain pitas and tortillas made from whole corn, which is a member of the whole-grain family.

## now can i have some alcohol?

I haven't included an "alcohol allowance" on this plan because alcohol isn't essential for health, and research shows that even moderate drinking—one drink a day—can increase the risk of breast cancer. But if you decide that you don't want to give up your occasional glass of wine, Belgian beer, or cocktail, I have suggestions for keeping your alcohol intake in balance. First, try to avoid alcohol until you've completed the thirty-day Cinch! plan, and from day thirty-one and beyond, limit yourself to once a week (maybe Saturday night) and stick to the Dietary Guidelines rule of no more than one drink per day for women and two for men. One drink equals a 5-ounce glass of wine, a 12-ounce beer, or a shot of liquor. Each provides about the same amount of alcohol and roughly 100 calories, but mixed drinks tend to pack the highest calorie punch due to mixers. To keep your calories in check, choose a flavor-infused, all-natural seltzer instead of the sugary stuff. Or stick with either a small glass of wine or one beer so that mixers aren't an issue. Sip it slowly, and then switch over to water with lemon or lime.

# 11

`24 25 26 27 28 29 30 31 32 33`

# cinch! goes the distance

ongratulations on completing the plan! This is a big achievement; you should feel incredibly proud. I hope you have reached your weight goal and experienced that "Yes!" moment. If you have more weight to lose, you now know that you can be successful, and you should continue to follow the plan. And if you have reached your goal weight, you should continue the plan to maintain your results. That's the beauty of Cinch! You may start at a different weight than someone else using this plan, but Cinch! is designed to help anyone achieve a healthy weight. The quiz on pages 154–56 is particularly important for understanding how you may need to modify Cinch! to meet your body's needs, but the goal for every reader is the same: to create an eating plan that will get you to and keep you at your goal weight. The closer you get to your goal, the slower your rate of weight loss will be (see page 250), but with Cinch!, there is no maintenance phase. Because Cinch! provides optimum nutrition for your body, you will be able to keep the weight off as long as you follow the plan. You have the blueprint you need, and the tools that you learned in chapter 6 taught you how to create your own meals so even if you've made every meal in this book, you'll never run out of new options. Your job now is to stay on track. That's why in this chapter I've laid out the eight most important strategies for doing just that!

I encourage you to begin using them immediately. As you move forward, these tried-and-true strategies can help you let go of your old habits (or lack of habits) and embrace the Cinch! way of eating for life.

I selected each strategy based on my nearly two decades of experience counseling my clients one-on-one as well as on the thoughts and feedback from real women featured in this book who have followed the Cinch! plan. Read through each strategy and start putting it into action today!

> 24 25 26 27 28 29 30
>
> I really am trying to pay attention to my hunger cues and how I feel before and after I eat.... This plan has been a real awakening to my body and mind.
>
> I AURENE, AGE 36

## strategy 1: plan ahead

Planning your meals—your foods, your portion sizes, and your meal times—is absolutely critical to your success. When you leave these things to chance, you're far more likely to skip meals, eat too much, or miss out on important nutrients that keep your body balanced, without cravings. Meal planning doesn't have to take a lot of time, but it does have to become a part of your daily routine.

At the end of the day, think through the next day. Go over your schedule and determine when you can eat, what you'd like to eat, and how to get it. If your kitchen is fully stocked, you may be good to go. When you have the ingredients you need on hand, you've overcome the first hurdle. But if that's not the case, you need to schedule a trip to the store into your day. And if you take your meals to work, you need to plan for that preparation.

A lot of my clients eat breakfast at home, pack their lunch and snack meals, and stop at the market on the way home from work to shop for the ingredients they need for dinner and the next day's lunch and snack. I live within walking distance of a few markets, so my shopping trip is as much a part of my daily routine as taking a shower. Others prefer sitting down on Sunday morning to plan out meals for the week and making one big trip to the supermarket.

If you know you'll be dining out, check out the menu ahead of time, which is easy to do since most restaurants post their menus online. You can decide what you'll order before you go. Don't be afraid to call in advance to ask for a special meal. Most restaurants are extremely accommodating to special dietary needs these days. And if you know that you won't be able to get the full "puzzle," eat the pieces you don't think you can get either before you go or after you get home. For example, at most restaurants it's easy to find a salad topped with grilled chicken with oil and vinegar on the side, which fills your produce, lean-protein, fat, and SASS pieces. But if the restaurant doesn't serve whole grains, eat one serving of whole-grain crackers before dinner (which can also help you avoid the bread basket) or three cups of popped popcorn when you get home. I love the Bearitos brand of microwave no-oil, no-salt organic popcorn for convenience, plus it doesn't require using oil, so you can "spend" your plant-based fat on another option. It's ideal to eat all five pieces of the puzzle at the same time, but having one or two pieces within a couple hours of the rest is a much better option than missing that important piece of your plan or eating something you don't want to eat.

The bottom line is when you've taken the time to think through your day and how to meet your needs, you are in the driver's seat. If you've ever gone camping, you've probably taken the time to think through everything you needed: sleeping bag, check; bug spray, check; mallet to pitch tent, check . . . And if you've ever been on vacation only to realize that you forgot something important and you find that it's not easy to replace (like your birth control!), you know how it can throw a wrench in your plans. When I taught at the University of South Florida, I had a student who went on a trip the week before finals and forgot her notes. I felt for her, but I couldn't allow her to reschedule. We all slip up sometimes, but the best way to avoid those moments of regret is to have a plan and stick with it. Make losing weight a priority. My clients tell me (and I feel the same) that when they plan ahead and stay on track, they feel better inside and out; they feel confident, successful, energized—a word that comes up often is "light"—in a nutshell, it's time and energy well spent. (See tips on pages 276–78 about surviving parties and about staying on track while traveling.)

*Action Plan:* If you struggle to find time to plan meals, use the time tracker on pages 244–45 to carve out time for planning your meals. You can use it not only to find time to walk or be active but also to create a schedule for preplanning your meals. Once you get into the groove, I think you'll welcome this extra daily "me time."

## strategy 2: stick to a schedule

As you read in chapter 7, the timing of your meals is a vital part of this plan. One of my clients started out eating breakfast at 8:00 A.M., lunch at noon, the snack at 4:00 P.M., dinner at 8:00 P.M., and the chocolate escape at 10:00 P.M.; perfect timing. She was steadily losing pounds and inches—until her weight loss suddenly slowed to a crawl. She was eating the same meals, but she had fallen in love with a particular snack—parfaits made with nonfat Greek yogurt, oats, fruit, nuts, and spices. She enjoyed them so much that she started eating her snack as a dessert right after dinner. That meant she went eight hours without eating and ate two meals as well as the chocolate escape all within a three-hour block. I reminded her that each meal is designed to fuel and nourish her body in the hours to come. By going long stretches without food, she was likely slowing down her metabolism, then filling the tank at night before her least active time of day. Her body couldn't retroactively use that fuel, and because it wasn't needed all at once, her glorious parfait was probably getting diverted to her fat cells. When she returned to her previous eating schedule, the pounds started coming off again, and she realized how much better she felt. Her mood was more stable, her digestive health was more regular, her afternoon slump disappeared, and her hunger was under control. If the importance of meal timing doesn't seem intuitive, this is one way to think about it: it's important for nutrients to show up when the work needs to get done. Not eating when you need food and overeating later is a lot like a quarter of the players on a football team showing up after the game has been played!

*Action Plan:* Think of your day in four blocks, each lasting three to five hours. If you work traditional hours, think of it this way: Block one is wake-up time through lunch; block two, lunch through midafternoon; block three, midafternoon to early evening; block four, early evening through bedtime. Eat one meal within each block, including breakfast within one hour of waking up. Even if you can't eat meals at exactly the same time every day, commit to eating them within the given block.

## strategy 3: measure!

I've been a nutritionist for nearly twenty years, and I still use measuring cups and spoons, especially for foods like olive oil, nuts and nut butters, and whole grains. When you eyeball it, it's easy to be off, and miscalculating by a little can make a big difference over time. Underestimating the veggies you eat by 20 percent isn't a big deal because most vegetables are so low in calories; maybe you'll stay two pounds heavier. But a 20 percent misjudgment on a portion of wild rice, whole-wheat pasta, or fruit can be enough to keep an extra thirty pounds on your frame!

So, make measuring a standard part of meal prep when you're at home. At a restaurant it's not practical (or cool) to whip out measuring cups, but the more you measure at home the more familiar you'll be with portion sizes and the more accurately you can judge just how much brown rice to eat or how much guacamole to spoon on top of your taco salad. My years of measuring at home have given me the confidence to better recognize portion sizes when I'm on the go.

*Action Plan:* Leave your measuring cups and spoons out on the countertop so you won't forget to use them. I have a few extra sets so I can leave them in various containers. I stash a quarter cup in my oatmeal canister, a tablespoon in my sliced-almonds container, and a half cup in the premade dish of whole grains I keep in the fridge.

A trick for traveling with food is to buy sealable containers that hold the perfect portion. I keep nuts in a condiment container that holds exactly two tablespoons, and I have others that are the perfect size for one serving of on-the-go foods like popcorn and dried fruit. That means I never have to worry about mindlessly overeating.

## strategy 4: separate the physical from the emotional

As I mentioned in chapter 2, practically from birth we're all taught to eat emotionally. We use food to celebrate, reward, and comfort one another and ourselves, and we get programmed to eat because food is available or we're bored or anxious. Cinch! helps you break this cycle by programming your body to experience mild to moderate physical hunger four times each day. Even if you wouldn't describe yourself as an emotional eater, the tools in chapter 8 can help you tease out body hunger from mind hunger. Recognizing the difference is the foundation of changing your relationship with food. In fact, focusing on that distinction alone has helped many of my clients lose weight.

Recognizing your thoughts in addition to your feelings is also key. In one recent study, Australian researchers found that the strength of food cravings was linked to how vividly people imagined a food. In one experiment, volunteers were asked to think about chocolate and then solve math questions, but they were so distracted, they took longer to solve math problems and weren't able to recall as much info. But when they were asked to form nonfood images in their minds, like a rainbow, or recall nonfood smells, such as eucalyptus, the cravings subsided. The more you raise the antenna on your awareness, the easier it is to filter out what your body really needs from what your mind wants, which is often just a short-lived coping mechanism that leaves you feeling worse in the end.

*Action Plan:* Start using a food diary. You can use one I coauthored called *The Ultimate Diet Log,* but even a simple notebook will suffice. Record not only what, when, and how much you ate, but also your thoughts, feelings, and physical signs of hunger and fullness. Tracking these at every meal, even for just one week, can help you identify important patterns, such as thinking about food when you're bored. Keeping a diary has helped many of my clients realize that they were eating whenever food was offered to them, even if they had just eaten an hour ago. This kind of insight is the key to transforming your relationship with food forever.

## strategy 5: select four to eight foolproof meals

When you're tired or busy you often make unwise choices. To give yourself a foolproof backup, choose one or two quick and easy go-to choices within each meal category (breakfast, lunch, dinner, and snack) with ingredients you can stock up on. (This strategy is like having that one perfect outfit tucked away in your closet.) Or preselect a few restaurant meals that fit the puzzle principle. In chapter 6, you'll find a list of restaurant meals that solve the puzzle, including meals at common chains like Chipotle and P. F. Chang's. Chipotle has been my personal savior on many occasions, and I know exactly what I'm going to order before I walk through the door.

My favorite breakfast backup is a slice of whole-grain toast (I keep

## what to do if you're tempted to get off track

Recently one of my clients "confessed" about an incident she was beating herself up over. She woke up early to go to the gym, ate a healthy breakfast and lunch, and felt amazingly confident and energized all day. That afternoon, her office celebrated a co-worker's birthday with cupcakes. She knew that one cupcake could cancel out most of her efforts for the day, but her internal dialogue said, "But they're red velvet, my favorite!" and she gave in. She felt awful, but I knew her well and in my opinion her indulgence had nothing to do with a lack of willpower. Diving into that cupcake was about not wanting to miss out on something she knew she would enjoy. Unfortunately, after she ate the cupcake she realized that the feeling she enjoyed more was being on track, not because the cupcake was "bad" or evil, but because afterward she felt sluggish, bloated, and unnourished. She said, "It was more than the weight. I felt like I wasn't taking good care of myself. I realized how good it feels to take care of myself!" Insights like this are powerful.

*The Strategy:* When you're facing the proverbial fork in the road (should I or shouldn't I), ask yourself two questions:

1.  If I give in and go off track, what will I be giving up that's important to me? Focus on feelings, not just results. In other words, even if your splurge didn't result in any weight gain, how might it affect your feelings of confidence, health (mental and physical), and energy?
2.  If I say no and stay on track, will I regret it an hour from now, tomorrow, or a week from now?

There are no right or wrong answers. Sometimes a few bites of dessert may feel like the right choice. But thinking these questions through can help you sort out your feelings in an honest, open way that allows your choices to reflect what's truly important to you.

## party survival skills

Between birthdays and anniversaries, the Super Bowl and the winter holidays, there's no doubt that you have many parties in your future. Use these five tips to stay on track while you celebrate with your friends, family, and co-workers:

1.  Eat before you drink. If you decide to have a cocktail, eat at least half of your meal first. Without food in your stomach, alcohol gets absorbed quickly, which means it will hit your brain in less than five minutes. And alcohol can not only lower your inhibitions but also up your appetite. Make your first few bites protein and fat. Both get emptied from your stomach slower, creating a better buffer for alcohol. Also, alternate sips of water with your beer, wine, or spirits.

2.  Scan your options before you act. If you're at a buffet, you're much more likely to overeat. A study from Penn State University found that when people were given more options they ate 43 percent more over the course of an hour. To curb your inclination to try a little of everything, look over all of the food first and then decide what fits your Cinch! strategy.

3.  Bring a "safety" dish. If you aren't sure you'll be able to meet your needs, bring a dish to share that fills the bill. A veggie tray with guacamole for dipping is a great choice because it's not unusual party fare and it can fill the veggie, plant-based-fat, and SASS pieces of your puzzle.

4.  Turn away from the table. Research studies show that the visibility and accessibility of food greatly impacts how much you'll eat. One study found that in a cafeteria, people bought more ice cream simply when the lid of the cooler was left open. Another showed that people given a sandwich in a transparent wrap ate more than those given sandwiches wrapped in opaque paper. Out of sight, out of mind really does hold true, so it's smart not only to stand away from the buffet table, but also to keep food out of your line of vision.

5.  Dress for awareness. Whether it's a clingy dress, slim-fitting pants, a belt, or a body shaper, constricting clothing can definitely prevent you from overdoing it. When fully expanded, your stomach can hold about six cups of food (think six baseballs!), so an antiexpansion strategy is a smart strategy for helping you stay in touch with your hunger meter.

a loaf stored in the freezer at all times) spread with two tablespoons of almond butter and a smoothie made from one cup of soy milk (I keep a shelf-stable container as backup in the cupboard), frozen blueberries (also a staple in my freezer), and ground cinnamon. The ingredients don't spoil quickly, and it takes less than five minutes to prepare.

*Action Plan:* Look through the meals in chapter 4 and the restaurant choices on pages 152–53 and create a short list of foolproof options. Write your restaurant choices on a sticky note or the back of a business card and stick it in your wallet, or post a note or photo of the meal on your fridge. Create a shopping list, and commit to staying stocked up on the ingredients.

## strategy 6: keep emergency backups with you at all times

This is a biggie! We all have days when life just doesn't proceed according to plan. Once I was stuck at the Charles De Gaulle Airport in Paris for hours on end. There was plenty of food available, but few healthy choices. Fortunately, I'd packed extra "kits" with me (see chapter 6): Just Tomatoes, Etc. dried crunchy carrot bits and dried organic soy nuts, Doctor Kracker crackers, and Justin's nut butter. By the second go-round I was desperately craving fresh food, but when I weighed my options I thought, okay, what's worse—eating an identical meal of snacks that fit the meal puzzle, or eating a heavy meal that'll leave me feeling sluggish and bloated? Staying on track felt like a smarter choice (it actually helped me sleep better on the plane). Best of all, I had a choice rather than being at the mercy of airport food.

Keeping a backup kit also comes in handy when you need to fill a piece of the puzzle. One of my clients has used this trick many times. If she gets stuck at work and the staff orders dinner in, she'll get grilled chicken and steamed veggies and fill the other pieces with her stash of sliced almonds, whole-grain crackers, and salt-free seasonings.

## stay on track when you travel

I have racked up a lot of frequent-flyer miles over the years, so I know firsthand that healthy eating can be a major challenge when traveling. But no matter what my schedule involves, I almost never veer from the Cinch! plan. If I do, I really feel it. My energy level plummets, my hunger gets thrown off, I tend to get run-down, and I have a tougher time maintaining my weight. So, I created a three-step, stay-on-track strategy that I put into action even before I pull out my suitcase:

1. The first thing I do is look through my entire travel itinerary and think through each and every meal. If my options may not include much in the way of fruits, veggies, and whole grains, I bring what I need to fill in the gaps, including unsweetened, preservative-free dried fruit like dried figs, or fresh fruit if possible (prewashed grapes), whole-grain crackers, prepopped popcorn, and dried veggies.

2. I go online to check the "healthy food radius" around my hotel, including grocery stores or food markets within walking distance.

3. Once I get to my destination, I stock my room with extras. On one recent trip, I knew that Whole Foods was a short walk from my hotel. Before I even unpacked my laptop, I headed over and bought fresh berries and baby carrots. I brought them to the conference center the next day in case I needed to fill a gap. One evening at a work-related dinner, I happily skipped the white rice that came with my meal knowing I wouldn't go to bed starving because I had healthy whole grains waiting for me in my room from the stash I packed.

These steps are a bit of extra work, but they lead you to the body you've always wanted. If you travel often, make backup foods part of your packing plan. They're just as essential as packing your toothbrush!

*Action Plan:* Review the options on pages 156–58. Add them to your grocery list or place an order online so you'll be good to go, then stash the items where you might need them, like your purse, desk drawer at work, or gym bag.

## strategy 7: banish negative self-talk

One of my favorite phrases is "I am continually a work in progress." Nobody is perfect, and sometimes we're too darned hard on ourselves! As I mentioned in chapter 8, negative self-talk can lead to negative emotions, which can trigger depression or cause you to want to punish yourself or cope in an unhealthy way. And that will work against you both physically and emotionally.

Sometimes the negativity really kicks in after a slipup, even if it's unintentional. I once had a client who realized after about a week that she was using a half-cup measuring cup for dry oats instead of a quarter-cup measuring cup. She was furious with herself and said, "I'm so stupid." Hearing comments like that breaks my heart because this plan is all about a better quality of life. When you talk to yourself in a punitive, judgmental way, you feel dejected rather than empowered, and that can lead to throwing in the towel.

The truth is that any change is difficult, and changing your diet is one of the most challenging tasks anyone can take on. If you hit a speed bump here or there, don't beat yourself up. If you nibble a little too much before dinner or take an extra helping of chocolate chips and you find yourself saying, "I blew it," remember that this is a process, not a win-or-lose game. In fact, all-or-nothing thinking tends to backfire when it comes to your weight-loss results. Throughout my years counseling people, I've had many clients tell me they were "doing good all day," then "messed up" and wound up bingeing all night or even all weekend. When you have all-or-nothing thinking, sometimes even a taste of something that's not on your plan can open the overeating floodgates. If this tends to happen to you, try to put a slipup in perspective and move on. Being a little bit off will make a much smaller dent in your weight-loss results than a big binge.

*Action Plan:* At the end of each day, think about three things you feel proud of or that went well. Perhaps you created a new puzzle meal based on the formula in chapter 6 and loved it, stayed on track with your meal times, or recognized mind hunger and satisfied it without turning to food. The more you pat yourself on the back, the less likely you'll be to focus on the negative. And if something didn't go well, think about what you learned from it that will help you in the future.

## put your results in perspective

You may be the exact same height, weight, and age as a friend who is following this plan, but you might lose weight at a different rate. In many ways, pounds are unpredictable. When you step on the scale, you're not just measuring body fat. Your total body weight is made up of seven distinct things: (1) muscle; (2) bone; (3) organs, like your lungs, heart, and liver; (4) fluids, including blood; (5) body fat; (6) the waste inside your digestive tract you haven't yet eliminated; and (7) glycogen, the form of carbohydrate you sock away in your liver and muscles as a backup fuel. Because of all the variables, it's entirely possible to have lost body fat and see absolutely no difference on the scale, or even see an upward blip, because one of the other six components has increased. What's most important is your personal pattern. If you're losing body fat, which this plan is designed to do for you, you should see a progressive change in your body. Also keep in mind that a quarter pound of fat is the equivalent of a stick of butter, so even if that loss doesn't register on your scale, it can make a big difference in how you look and how your clothes fit!

## strategy 8: listen to your instincts

You know yourself better than anyone else, and your own insights are incredibly powerful. Let them guide you to let you know how you're doing and when you need more help or support from others. Communicating with yourself in an honest, open way will allow you to shine a light on your thoughts, feelings, and behaviors in a manner that gently examines where you are and where you want to be. In the big picture, this plan is about transforming your relationship with food, which includes the following:

1. Understanding the ideal amounts, combinations, and timing of meals to best support your body's healthy weight
2. Examining how your triggers about what, when, where, and how much to eat differ from the ideal
3. Creating new social and psychological patterns and coping mechanisms that will allow you to eat healthfully in a way that feels very intuitive and self-nurturing

*Action Plan:* You've probably been on a number of diets before. But Cinch! isn't a diet. It's a strategy. This thirty-day program is the training period for living a strategic lifestyle. The Wikipedia definition of strategic planning is "Defining [a] direction and making decisions [and] allocating... resources to pursue this strategy." By using all the tools in this book, that's exactly what you're doing. So start thinking of yourself as the captain of the ship. You're at the helm and only you can decide where you're going and how to get there. You have all the training and experience you need to take this journey. Enjoy your newfound food freedom and all that comes with it, including having the body you've dreamed of!

# acknowledgments

To everyone at HarperCollins: Thank you for welcoming me with open arms and giving me the opportunity to share my heart and soul with the world. And special thanks to my editor, Nancy Hancock, for your faith in my abilities, our heart-to-heart talks, your terrific sense of humor, and for allowing me to be me in the pages of this book.

My gratitude to Bill Stankey and Mary Lalli at Westport Entertainment; my attorney, Marc Chamlin, with Loeb & Loeb, and the amazing Marta Tracy of Marty Tracy Entertainment. Thank you for believing in me, Marta, and for your tireless, passionate work. You are colleague, friend, and family.

This book could not have come together without the talents and support of Stephanie Breakstone and Suzanne Scholsberg. I can't thank you enough for jumping into the trenches with me when I needed you. I hope you know how much I admire you both professionally and personally.

Thank you to the dietetic students and interns for volunteering your time and skills to help me with this project: Jamie Schottenfeld, Diane Blahut, Anita Mirchandani, and Anna-Lisa Finger. I have no doubt that each of you will succeed in anything you set out to do.

To all of my clients—thank you for putting your trust in me and making me feel like I have the best job in the world. And to the incredible women who made the commitment to formally test this eating plan, it was an honor and a privilege getting to know each of you. Your invaluable feedback and experiences have improved this book, and your stories are inspirational. I also want to thank Chad Tenorio for capturing the inner and outer beauty of each of these women in your photos.

Many thanks to everyone at *Shape* magazine, especially Valerie Latona, Trisha Calvo, Samantha Trenk, A. J. Hanley, Marty Munson, and Jane Seymour. I love being part of the *Shape* family. Thank you for partnering with me to share Cinch! success stories with your readers. I admire your commitment to helping women across the country live healthier, balanced lives.

Much appreciation to my colleagues who have always cheered me on and have become trusted friends, especially Dave Grotto, Tara Gidus, Mitzi Dulan, Jackie Newgent, Kate Gegan, Bonnie Taub-Dix, Alanna Levine, Christine Gerbstadt, Lisa Davis, and Amy Gorin, and especially to Rachel Metlzer Warren and Leah McLaughlin for your incredible gestures of support, generosity, and friendship. I'm so lucky to have you in my life.

To my parents, James and Carol Crowell, and every member of my Crowell, Sass, DeTota, and Salvagno families—I love you. And to my other wonderful friends in New York who encouraged and supported me every step of the way: Denise Maher, Michael Dolan, Ani Mozian-Whitney, Teresa Dumain, and the incredible James Corbett—thank you, James, for always being there and for never letting my spark go out!

And finally to my husband, Jack Bremen, and my beautiful sister, Diane Salvagno, to whom this book is dedicated. Jack you have *always* been there for me for everything and anything I have ever needed throughout this journey. Thank you for making me feel loved and for bringing out the best in me. And to Diane, I feel like I'm with you every day even though we live miles apart. Thank you for your unconditional love, support, friendship, and laughter.

# index

acetic acid, 76–77
acetylcholine, 47
ADI (Acceptable Daily Intake), 24–25
afterburn myth, 247
AGEs (advanced glycation end products), 209–10
albuminuria, 24
alcohol consumption, 26, 266–67
alkylamines, 83
almond butter, 42
almonds: Berry Almond French Toast, 99; Blueberry Smoothie with Almond Toast, 96; 5-Day Fast Forward meals with, 33–36; 5-Day Fast Forward plan use of, 30; Green Tea and Vanilla Banana Almond Smoothie, 103; grocery guidelines for, 31, 37; Mulberry Almond Parfait, 97; nutritional benefits of, 41–42; Pear Ginger Almond Pancakes, 101; Peppery Kiwi Almond Crunch, 104; Pineapple Almond Peppercorn Parfait, 112; Tangerine Almond Twist, 106; Vanilla Almond Frozen Banana, 115
Alzheimer's disease, 23, 85, 202
American Heart Association, 23
animal-based protein, 173
antibiotic-resistant salmonella, 94
antioxidants: catechins, 31; in cinnamon, 85; curcumin, 88; EGCG (epigallocatechin gallate), 32; flavonoids, 22, 140; isoflavones, 52, 54, 55; naringenin, 78–79; polyphenols, 22;

spinach as source of, 38; vitamin E, 42; weight-loss results of, 74–75
apples: Apple Pecan Breakfast Pilaf, 103; Cinnamon Walnut Apple Crisp, 107
artichokes, 166
artificial sweeteners, 24–26
Artisana, 42
avocados: Avocado Egg Dip, 111; Black Bean Tacos with Cilantro-Jalapeño Guacamole, 133; California Sunshine Salad, 113; Chilled Lentil and Wild Rice Salad, 132; Fish Tacos with Cilantro-Jalapeño Guacamole, 130; Green-Tea Chicken with Avocado Corn Salad, 120–21; Layered Bean Dip with Cilantro-Jalapeño Guacamole, 134; Mango Mint Avocado Smoothie, 106; Pineapple Avocado Tacos, 110; Spicy Avocado Tostadas, 119; Strawberry Avocado Tacos, 102–3; Tangerine Tofu Tacos with Cilantro-Jalapeño Guacamole, 114; Very Berry Omelet with Avocado Toast, 101; Zesty Bean and Summer Slaw Pita, 135

Balsamic Truffles, 146
Banana Hazelnut Ricotta Toast, 98
beans, 177
belly fat, 76, 210
Berry Almond French Toast, 99
beverages: alcohol, 26, 266–67; Cinch! options for, 20–21, 92–93; coffee, 21, 32; 5-Day Fast Forward plan, 32; water, 34;

beverages *(continued)*
   Zesty Cinnamon Basil Berry Tea, 21–22,
      32, 93
bifidobacterium, 49
Black Bean Tacos with Cilantro-Jalapeño
   Guacamole, 133
Black and Blue Salad, 117
Black Currant Crunch, 98
black pepper, health benefits of, 84
bloating, 254–55
blueberries: Blueberry Smoothie with
   Almond Toast, 96; Dark Chocolate
   Oatmeal with a Side of Minted Blueberry
   Yogurt, 101; health benefits of, 85;
   Herbed Popcorn with a Blueberry
   Coconut Smoothie, 114
BMI (body mass index), 200
body: Cinch! plan for reconnecting with
   your, 17, 20; 5-Day Fast Forward plan
   and resetting your, 57–61
BPA (bisphenol A), 209, 211
bread selection, 263–64
breakfast recipes: dairy meals, 96–99; egg
   meals, 99–101; vegan meals, 101–4;
   Zero-Prep Cinch! core meal kits, 158
Breakfast Tacos with Fresh Figs, 100
breast cancer, 26, 94, 266
Broiled Grapefruit with Herbed Feta, 107
B vitamins, 42

caffeine, 141
California Chicken Cilantro Burrito
   Bowl, 123
California Harvest Pita with Minted
   Yogurt, 102
California Sunshine Salad, 113
calories: fat as percentage of, 174–75, 177–
   79; SASS used to cut down, 73–74; why
   calorie counting is outdated, 191–93;
   why they are not created equal, 189–91.
   *See also* weight loss
cancers: breast, 26, 94, 266; colorectal, 40,
   94; eating fruit to reduce risk of, 161;
   risks associated with, 23, 177; squamous-
   cell carcinoma skin, 79; turmeric as
   fighting, 85
capsaicin, 43, 81–82
carbohydrate-protein ratio, 207–9
carb-rich foods, 170, 198–99
catechins, 31

cells: fueling your, 190; life-span of, 199
Cherry Almond Green Tea Smoothie, 104
chicken lunch/dinner recipes: California
   Chicken Cilantro Burrito Bowl, 123;
   Chicken Pesto Pita, 121; Chicken
   Satay Pita, 123; Chilled Brown Rice
   and Vegetable Salad with Brazil Nut–
   Dusted Chicken, 122; Chilled Herbed
   Chicken Pasta Salad, 121; Garlicky
   Barley Vegetable Chicken Soup, 123;
   Green-Tea Chicken with Avocado
   Corn Salad, 120–21; Mediterranean
   Broccoli Couscous Platter, 122; Spinach,
   Artichoke, and Olive Chicken Pasta,
   121; Wild Rice and Chicken Lettuce
   Wraps with Citrus Slaw, 122
Chickpea and Red Quinoa Lettuce
   Wraps, 134
Chilled Brown Rice and Vegetable Salad
   with Brazil Nut–Dusted Chicken, 122
Chilled Lentil and Wild Rice Salad, 132
Chipotle Restaurant, 152
chocolate: benefits of eating, 140–41, 144–
   46; Chocolate Pear Ginger Smoothie,
   96–97, 146; Dark Chocolate Oatmeal
   with a Side of Minted Blueberry Yogurt,
   101; Fair Trade, 144; food cravings and,
   137–38; history of, 139; rules for eating,
   138–39
chocolate-chip exercise, 230–32, 234
Chocolate Escape recipes: Balsamic Truffles,
   146; Citrus Zest Truffles, 147; Green Tea
   Truffles, 148; Peppercorn Truffles, 148;
   Spicy Chipotle Truffles, 147
cholesterol: eggs and, 46, 48; HDL, 145,
   174, 211; LDL, 42, 105, 141, 145, 174,
   211; slashing your, 174
choline, 47
Cinch! Caesar Salad, 118
Cinch! meals: Chocolate Escape, 137, 146–
   48; eating like clockwork rule on, 12;
   exclusion of red meat in, 93–95; 5-Day
   Fast Forward, 15, 33–36; 5-Piece Puzzle
   of, 12–13, 90–92; foods included in, 93;
   making flavor the focus of, 13; "puzzle
   principle" used for, 95–96; variety of,
   13–14; Zero-Prep Cinch! core meal kits,
   156–58, 277–78. *See also* Cinch! recipes
Cinch! Picnic Snack, 113
Cinch! plan: beverages options in the,

20–26; compared to *Flat Belly Diet!*, 4; exercise component of, 235–48; 5-Day Fast Forward option of the, 14–16; 5-Piece Puzzle foundation of, 12–13, 90–92; general overview of the, 2–5; getting off track, 253–54, 275; indulging in a splurge during, 251–52; power of the structure of, 17; put your results in perspective, 281; reconnecting with your body through the, 17, 20; as "retrotarian" diet, 95; reviewing the twenty-five-day plan rules of the, 11–14; strategies for success with the, 268–81; unique characteristics of, 6

Cinch! plan questions: on alcohol, 26, 266–67; grocery-related, 260–66; on personal health, 257–60; on weight loss, 249–57

Cinch! plan rules: 1: Eat Like Clockwork, 12; 2: Think, "Five Pieces Four Times a Day," 12–13; 3: Make Flavor Your Focus, 13

Cinch! plan strategies: 1: plan ahead, 269–71; 2: stick to a schedule, 271–72; 3: measure, 272–73; 4: separate the physical from emotional, 273–74; 5: select 4-8 foolproof meals, 274, 277; 6: emergency backups, 156–58, 277–78; 7: banish negative self-talk, 279–80; 8: listen to your instincts, 280–81

Cinch! recipes: breakfast meals, 96–104; Chocolate Escape, 146–48; egg meals, 111–12; 5-Day Fast Forward meals, 33–36; lunch and dinner meals, 117–36; snacks, 104, 106–7, 110; vegan snacks, 112–15; Zero-Prep Cinch! core meal kits, 158. *See also* Cinch! meals

cinnamon: Cinnamon Cherry Yogurt with Peanut Butter Crackers, 115; Cinnamon Walnut Apple Crisp, 107; health benefits of, 84, 85; Zesty Cinnamon Basil Berry Tea, 21–22, 32, 93

circle of sustainability, 25

citrus juice/zest: Citrus Salmon Salad, 129; Citrus Zest Truffles, 147; health benefits of SASS category of, 70, 77–79, 184; listed types of, 182; Savory Spaghetti Squash with Citrus Zest, 120; Zesty Cinnamon Basil Berry Tea, 21–22, 32. *See also* SASS (Slimming And Satiating Seasonings)

coconut oil, 145

coconut yogurt, 30, 50, 51

coffee, 21, 32

collagen, 43

colorectal cancer, 40, 94

CPFs (chlorphyrifos), 202

Cranberry Cashew Parfait, 103

Cranberry Parmesan Herbed Popcorn, 107

Cranberry Pesto Egg Spread, 112

Cranberry Walnut Quinoa Pilaf, 100

CRP (C-reactive protein), 141, 144

curcumin, 88

dairy breakfast recipes: Banana Hazelnut Ricotta Toast, 98; Black Currant Crunch, 98; Blueberry Smoothie with Almond Toast, 96; Chocolate Pear Ginger Smoothie, 96–97, 146; Mulberry Almond Parfait, 97; Raspberry Brazil Nut Pita, 99; Spicy Grape Parfait, 98; Strawberry Cardamom Smoothie with Cashew Oatmeal, 97; Strawberry Green Tea Muesli, 99; Zesty Cranberry Walnut Parfait, 97

dairy lunch/dinner recipes: Black and Blue Salad, 117; Cinch! Caesar Salad, 118; Fresh Mozzarella Basil "Pizzalad," 119; Herbed Walnut Artichoke Lettuce Wraps, 120; Mediterranean Pasta Salad, 119; Ricotta Primavera Penne, 118; Savory Spaghetti Squash with Citrus Zest, 120; Smoked Gouda and Grilled Onion Salad, 117; Spicy Avocado Tostadas, 119; Spinach Walnut Feta Pita, 118

dairy snack recipes: Broiled Grapefruit with Herbed Feta, 107; Cinnamon Walnut Apple Crisp, 107; Cranberry Parmesan Herbed Popcorn, 107; Mango Mint Avocado Smoothie, 106; Peppery Kiwi Almond Crunch, 104; Peppery Pear Crunch, 110; Pineapple Avocado Tacos, 110; Sonoma Snack, 106; Strawberry Vanilla Hazelnut "Ice Cream," 110; Tangerine Almond Twist, 106

Dark Chocolate Oatmeal with a Side of Minted Blueberry Yogurt, 101

dating issues, 260

diet chaos: associated with being overweight or obese, 6–7; definition of, 9; ending the, 7, 10 diet soda, 24–26

Digging Deeper grid, 226–27

dinner recipes: chicken meals, 120–23; dairy meals, 117–20; seafood meals, 128–31; turkey meals, 124–27; vegan meals, 132–36; Zero-Prep Cinch! core meal kits, 158

dried fruit, 161, 164

eating patterns: eating slowly to eat less, 135; emotional eating, 6–7, 10, 66, 213–34; Insighter Questions assessing your, 62, 64–68; type 2 diabetes and associated, 40. *See also* healthy eating

Eat Like Clockwork rule, 12

*E. coli* outbreaks, 95

Edamame Cashew ginger Stir-Fry, 133

EGCG (epigallocatechin gallate), 32

egg meals: Avocado Egg Dip, 111; Berry Almond French Toast, 99; Breakfast Tacos with Fresh Figs, 100; Cranberry Pesto Egg Spread, 112; Cranberry Walnut Quinoa Pilaf, 100; Fig and Olive Snack, 111; Open-Faced Pesto Egg Sandwich, 111; Pesto Breakfast Pita, 100; Spicy Egg Tacos with Cilantro-Jalapeño Guacamole, 112; Very Berry Omelet with Avocado Toast, 101

eggs. *See* organic eggs

emergency backup kits, 156–58, 277–78

emotional eating: chocolate-chip exercise for examining, 230–32, 234; Digging Deeper grid, 226–27; finding alternatives to, 218–26; Food and Feelings grid on, 222, 223; getting individualized help for, 217; how your relationship impacts your, 232–33; Insighter Question assessing your, 66; learning to conquer, 6–7; pattern of, 10; phenomenon of, 213–18; unlearning, 226–29. *See also* foods

emotional symptoms, 224–26

exercise. *See* walking

Fair Trade chocolate, 144

family farms, 206

fats: fully hydrogenated oil, 179–80; margarine, corn oil, and PUFAs, 180–81; as percentage of calories, 174–75, 177–79; plant-based, 90, 150, 152–53, 173–76, 186; saturated, 94, 176–80; solid versus liquid, 178; trans-fat, 176–79

Federation of American Societies for Experimental Biology (FASEB) journal, 85

feelings: connections between foods and, 215–18; emotional symptoms of, 224–26; Food and Feelings grid, 222, 223; how your relationship impacts weight and, 232–33

fiber, 171, 210

Fiesta Pasta Salad, 126

Fig and Olive Snack, 111

Fish Tacos with Cilantro-Jalapeño Guacamole, 130

5-Day Diary: days 1-5 in the, 64–68; Insighter Questions of, 62, 64–68; wrap-up of the, 69

5-Day Fast Forward meals: about the, 15; Parfait, 33; Salad, 34–35; Scramble, 33; Smoothie, 35–36

5-Day Fast Forward plan: assessing whether to use the, 15–16; description of, 11, 14–15; 5-Day Diary kept during, 61–69; grocery guidelines/list for, 31, 37; meals of the, 15, 33–36; nutritional benefits of the, 54–56; rules of the, 36; seasonings for the, 31–32; things to know before starting the, 29–30; three goals accomplished using the, 28–29; what you can expect during each day of, 56, 58–61

5-Piece Puzzle: Cheat Sheet for, 185–87; as Cinch! foundation, 12–13, 90–92; fruit as part of the, 90, 150, 151, 159–61, 164, 185; "Goldilocks" effect and serving sizes, 20, 151, 154–56, 252; lean protein as part of the, 90, 150, 152, 171–73, 186; meal ingredients using "puzzle principle," 95–96, 150–54; plant-based fat as part of the, 90, 150, 152–53, 173–76; restaurant meals, 152; SASS as part of the, 90, 150, 181–84, 187; vegetables as part of the, 90, 150, 151, 164–67, 185; whole grains as part of the, 90, 150, 151–52, 167–71, 185; Zero-Prep Cinch! core meal kits, 156–58, 277–78. *See also specific recipes*

*Flat Belly Diet!,* 3–4

flavonoids, 22, 140

food cravings, 137–38, 273–74

food diary: 5-Day Diary, 62, 64–69; keeping a, 274
Food and Feelings grid, 222, 223
foods: buying locally produced, 265; carb-rich, 170, 198–99; Cinch! meals included, 93; connections between feelings and, 215–18; folate-rich, 40; organic, 201–7; processed, 209–12; reduced-fat, 265–66; USDA-certified organic soy, 54, 55. See also emotional eating; grocery guidelines/list
free radicals, 105
freezing spinach and raspberries, 45
Fresh Mozzarella Basil "Pizzalad," 119
fruit: dried, 161, 164; as 5-Piece Puzzle piece, 90, 150, 151, 185; how to use for meals, 90, 150, 151, 159–61, 164
fully hydrogenated oil, 179–80

garlic: Garlicky Barley Vegetable Chicken Soup, 123; health benefits of, 84–85
getting off track, 253–54, 275
ginger: Chocolate Pear Ginger Smoothie, 96–97, 146; Edamame Cashew ginger Stir-Fry, 133; Ginger Turkey Stir-Fry, 127; Ginger Yogurt with Carambola Crunch, 115; health benefits of, 84; Pear Ginger Almond Pancakes, 101; Salmon Ginger Rice Bowl, 128
gingivitis, 50
glucose intolerance, 82
glycemic index, 159
GMOs (genetically modified organisms), 53, 54, 203
"Goldilocks" effect, 20, 151, 252
grapefruits, 160, 184
grapes: health benefits of, 105; Sonoma Snack, 106
Greek yogurt, 50
green tea: Cherry Almond Green Tea Smoothie, 104; Green-Tea Chicken with Avocado Corn Salad, 120–21; Green Tea Truffles, 148; Green Tea and Vanilla Banana Almond Smoothie, 103; health benefits of, 22, 31, 32; Strawberry Green Tea Muesli, 99. See also teas
grilling tips, 264–65
grocery guidelines/list: almonds/almond butter, 31, 37, 42; Cinch! plan questions related to, 260–66; organic eggs, 31, 37,
47–48; raspberries, 31, 37; yogurt, 31, 37, 50–52. See also foods
ground turkey, 266

HDL cholesterol, 145, 174, 211
health ratings, 67
healthy eating: assessing motivation for, 68; 5-Day Fast Forward plan benefits for, 54–56; Mediterranean style of eating as, 94, 95; nutrient balance for, 196–98. See also eating patterns
heart disease, 23
Herbed Popcorn with a Blueberry Coconut Smoothie, 114
Herbed Turkey and spinach "Spaghetti" Bake, 126
Herbed Walnut Artichoke Lettuce Wraps, 120
herbs/spices: health benefits of, 70, 84–85, 88–89; listed types of, 182–83; R.W. Knudsen's Organic Mulling Spices, 81; storing, 88
high blood pressure, 23, 144
homocysteine, 47
hot peppers: health benefits of, 80–82; listed types of, 182; as SASS category, 70
hunger: description of, 17; "Goldilocks" outcome of, 20, 151, 252; learning to monitor your, 17, 20; oleoylethanolamide as curbing, 36
hydrogen sulfide, 49

immune system: raspberries building up the, 44; tea benefits for, 83–84; vitamin A benefits for, 38, 40
infertility, 177
Insighter Questions: description of, 62; in 5-Day Diary, 64–68
isoflavones, 52, 54, 55

ketones, 43
kidney disease, 24

lactobacillus, 49
lauric acid, 145
Layered Bean Dip with Cilantro-Jalapeño Guacamole, 134
LDL cholesterol, 42, 105, 141, 145, 174, 211
lean protein: animal-based, 173; beans as source of, 177; carbohydrate ratio

lean protein *(continued)*
  to, 207–9; as 5-Piece Puzzle piece, 90,
  150, 152, 186; plant-based, 172–73;
  suggestions for using, 171–73
Lemon Thyme Scallops, 130–31
liposuction, 255–56
low-sodium diet, 257–58
Loyola University Health System, 24
lunch recipes: chicken meals, 120–23; dairy
  meals, 117–20; seafood meals, 128–31;
  turkey meals, 124–27; vegan meals, 132–
  36; Zero-Prep Cinch! core meal kits, 158

magnesium, 42, 44
Make Flavor Your Focus rule, 13
Mango Mint Avocado Smoothie, 106
Mara Natha, 42
meals. *See* Cinch! meals
Mediterranean Broccoli Couscous
  Platter, 122
Mediterranean Lentils over Couscous, 132
Mediterranean Minted Turkey Salad, 125
Mediterranean Pasta Salad, 119
Mediterranean Shrimp Pizza, 129
Mediterranean style of eating, 94, 95
men: fluid requirements of, 34; helping
  them to lose weight, 256–57; red meat
  intake and health risk of, 94
mercury contamination, 259, 262–63
metabolic syndrome, 78
metabolism: afterburn myth on exercise
  and, 247; regular meals to regulate your,
  192–93; water relationship to regulating,
  35. *See also* weight loss
milk buying tips, 264
mini mental vacations, 228–29
Mulberry Almond Parfait, 97
"My Size" quiz, 154–56
My Stories: Adina Friedman, 56–57; Cat
  Chez, 142–43; Heidi Matzelle, 86–87;
  Jennifer Steinruck, 220–21; Maleika
  Cole, 194–95; Miri Frankel, 108–9; Sally
  Andrea, 162–63; Selena Shepps, 18–19

NAFLD (nonalcoholic fatty liver
  disease), 24
naringenin, 78–79
negative self-talk, 279–80
*nigari,* 54
nutrient balance, 196–98

oleic acid, 36
oleoylethanolamide, 36
Open-Faced Pesto Egg Sandwich, 111
organic eggs: cholesterol and, 46, 48; 5-Day
  Fast Forward meals with, 33–35; 5-Day
  Fast Forward plan use of, 30; grocery
  guidelines for, 31, 37, 47–48; nutritional
  benefits of, 45–48
organic foods: economic purchase of,
  205–6; health benefits of, 201–5; USDA
  certified organic label of, 207; USDA-
  certified organic soy foods, 54, 55
overweight/obesity: belly fat and, 76, 210;
  diet chaos associated with, 6–7; glucose
  intolerance associated with, 82; how
  your relationship impacts your, 232–33;
  psychological stress and, 61; studies on
  future trends of, 3

Panera Bread Restaurant, 153
Parfait time: 5-Day Diary on, 64–68;
  5-Day Fast Forward, 33
party survival skills, 276
Peanut Butter Blackberry Toast, 102
Peanut Butter Mulberry Toast, 104
Peanut Butter Plum Toast, 113
Pear Ginger Almond Pancakes, 101
Peppercorn Truffles, 148
Peppers with Polenta and Pine Nuts, 136
Peppery Broad Beans over Vegetable
  Barley, 134
Peppery Kiwi Almond Crunch, 104
Peppery Pear Crunch, 110
personal health questions: on Cinch! plan
  and dating, 260; on Cinch! plan and
  low-sodium diet, 257–58; on taking
  supplements, 258–60. *See also* weight-
  loss questions
Pesto Breakfast Pita, 100
P.F. Chang Restaurant, 152
PFCs (polyfluoroalkyl chemicals), 210–11
phytochemical, 74
Pineapple Almond Peppercorn Parfait, 112
Pineapple Avocado Tacos, 110
plant-based fat: as 5-Piece Puzzle piece, 90,
  150, 152–53, 186; suggestions for using,
  173–76
plant-based protein, 172–73
plastic surgery, 255–56
polyphenols, 22

probiotics, 49, 258

processed foods, 209–12

produce: as 5-Piece Puzzle piece, 90, 150, 151, 185; fruit, 90, 150, 151, 159–61, 164, 185; vegetables, 90, 150, 151, 164–67, 185

protein. *See* lean protein

psychological stress, 61

PUFAs (polyunsaturated fatty acids), 180–81

raspberries: 5-Day Fast Forward meals with, 33–36; 5-Day Fast Forward plan use of, 30; freezing, 45; grocery guidelines for, 31, 37; nutritional benefits of, 42–44; Raspberry Brazil Nut Pita, 99; Raspberry Pistachio Cereal, 102

red meat, 93–95

reduced-fat foods, 265–66

relationships-weight-emotions link, 232–33

restaurant meals, 152–53

resveratrol, 105

"retrotarian" diet, 95

Ricotta Primavera Penne, 118

Romano's Macaroni Grill, 153

Ruby Tuesday, 153

rules: Cinch! plan, 12–13; 5-Day Fast Forward plan, 36

R.W. Knudsen's Organic Mulling Spices, 81

Salad Time: 5-Day Diary on, 64–68; 5-Day Fast Forward meal, 34–35

Salmon Ginger Rice Bowl, 128

SASS (Slimming And Satiating Seasonings): cutting back on sodium using, 72; description of, 12, 13, 70–71; 5-Day Fast Forward plan, 31–32, 37; as 5-Piece Puzzle piece, 90, 150, 153–54, 181–84, 187; grocery list for, 37; health benefits of, 71–75; herbs/spices category of, 70, 84–85, 88–89, 182–83; hot peppers category of, 70, 80–82, 182; superheroes among, 85; tea category of, 70, 82–84, 182; vinegar category of, 70, 75–77, 182. *See also* citrus juice/zest

saturated fat, 94, 176–80

Savory Spaghetti Squash with Citrus Zest, 120

Scramble meals: 5-Day Diary on, 64–68; 5-Day Fast Forward, 33

seafood lunch/dinner recipes: Citrus Salmon Salad, 129; Fish Tacos with Cilantro-Jalapeño Guacamole, 130; Lemon Thyme Scallops, 130–31; Mediterranean Shrimp Pizza, 129; mercury contamination concerns, 259, 262–63; Salmon Ginger Rice Bowl, 128; Shrimp Creole, 128–29; Shrimp Pesto Salad, 131; Sicilian Sardine Pasta, 131; Tuna Pecan Pasta, 130; Tuna-Stuffed Tomatoes, 128

seasonings. *See* SASS (Slimming And Satiating Seasonings)

self-talk: negative, 279–80; positive, 229

serving sizes: "Goldilocks" effect and, 20, 151, 252; "My Size" quiz for, 154–56; visualizing your, 154

Shrimp Creole, 128–29

Shrimp Pesto Salad, 131

Sicilian Sardine Pasta, 131

*skyr* yogurt, 50

Smell and Taste Treatment and Research Foundation, 74

Smoked Gouda and Grilled Onion Salad, 117

Smoothie time: 5-Day Diary on, 64–68; 5-Day Fast Forward meal, 35–36

snacks: Chocolate Escape, 146–48; dairy meal, 104, 106–7, 110; vegan, 112–15

soda: hazards of diet, 24–26; health problems associated with, 23–24

sodium reduction, 72, 257–58, 260–62

Sonoma Snack, 106

soy-based products: nutritional benefits of, 52, 54; as plant-based protein source, 172–73; safety of, 55; USDA-certified organic soy foods, 54, 55; as vegan substitute, 30, 50

spices. *See* herbs/spices

Spicy Avocado Tostadas, 119

Spicy Chipotle Truffles, 147

Spicy Egg Tacos with Cilantro-Jalapeño Guacamole, 112

Spicy Grape Parfait, 98

spinach: 5-Day Fast Forward meals with, 33–35; 5-Day Fast Forward plan use of, 30; freezing fresh, 45; frozen versus fresh, 39; grocery guidelines for, 31, 37; nutritional benefits of, 38, 40; Spinach, Artichoke, and Olive Chicken Pasta, 121; Spinach Walnut Feta Pita, 118

splurging tips, 251–52
Strawberry Avocado Tacos, 102–3
Strawberry Cardamom Smoothie with
    Cashew Oatmeal, 97
Strawberry Green Tea Muesli, 99
Strawberry Vanilla Hazelnut "Ice Cream," 110
Strawberry Walnut "Ice Cream" with Lime
    Zest, 114
stress, 61, 140
substitutions: making smart, 92; vegan
    yogurt, 30, 50, 51, 52, 54, 55; vegetarian
    yogurt, 30, 50
supplements, 258–60

Tangerine Almond Twist, 106
Tangerine Tofu Tacos with Cilantro-
    Jalapeño Guacamole, 114
teas: health benefits of, 70, 82–84; Zesty
    Cinnamon Basil Berry Tea, 21–22, 32,
    93. See also green tea
Think, "Five Pieces Four Times a Day" rule,
    12–13
tofu, 54
Tomato, Basil, and Walnut Salad with
    Cannellini Beans, 132
trans fat, 176–79
traveling strategies, 278
triglycerides, 51
Tuna Pecan Pasta, 130
Tuna-Stuffed Tomatoes, 128
turkey lunch/dinner recipes: Fiesta Pasta
    Salad, 126; Ginger Turkey Stir-Fry,
    127; Herbed Turkey and spinach
    "Spaghetti" Bake, 126; Mediterranean
    Minted Turkey Salad, 125; Turkey
    Almond Pita, 127; Turkey Mock Tacos,
    124; Turkey Pesto Salad, 126; Turkey
    Pita "Pizzalad," 124; Turkey Walnut
    Pita, 125; Turkey and Wild Rice—
    Stuffed Peppers, 125
Turkey Pesto Salad, 126
turmeric, 85, 88
2 percent milk, 264
type 2 diabetes: berries reducing risk of,
    44; eating patterns associated with, 40;
    liver fat marker for, 76; naringenin as
    preventive for, 78; sugar intake associated
    with, 23; trans fat risk for, 177

Vanilla Almond Frozen Banana, 115

vegan lunch/dinner recipes: Black
    Bean Tacos with Cilantro-Jalapeño
    Guacamole, 133; Chickpea and Red
    Quinoa Lettuce Wraps, 134; Chilled
    Lentil and Wild Rice Salad, 132;
    Edamame Cashew ginger Stir-Fry,
    133; Layered Bean Dip with Cilantro-
    Jalapeño Guacamole, 134; Mediterranean
    Lentils over Couscous, 132; Peppers with
    Polenta and Pine Nuts, 136; Peppery
    Broad Beans over Vegetable Barley, 134;
    Tomato, Basil, and Walnut Salad with
    Cannellini Beans, 132; Zesty Bean and
    Summer Slaw Pita, 135
vegan meals: Apple Pecan Breakfast Pilaf,
    103; California Harvest Pita with
    Minted Yogurt, 102; Cherry Almond
    Green Tea Smoothie, 104; Cranberry
    Cashew Parfait, 103; Dark Chocolate
    Oatmeal with a Side of Minted Blueberry
    Yogurt, 101; Green Tea and Vanilla
    Banana Almond Smoothie, 103; Peanut
    Butter Blackberry Toast, 102; Peanut
    Butter Mulberry Toast, 104; Pear Ginger
    Almond Pancakes, 101; Raspberry
    Pistachio Cereal, 102; Strawberry
    Avocado Tacos, 102–3
vegan snacks: California Sunshine
    Salad, 113; Cinch! Picnic Snack,
    113; Cinnamon Cherry Yogurt with
    Peanut Butter Crackers, 115; Ginger
    Yogurt with Carambola Crunch, 115;
    Herbed Popcorn with a Blueberry
    Coconut Smoothie, 114; Peanut Butter
    Plum Toast, 113; Pineapple Almond
    Peppercorn Parfait, 112; Strawberry
    Walnut "Ice Cream" with Lime Zest,
    114; Tangerine Tofu Tacos with
    Cilantro-Jalapeño Guacamole, 114;
    Vanilla Almond Frozen Banana, 115
vegan substitutions: coconut yogurt, 30, 50,
    51; soy-based products, 30, 50, 52, 54, 55
vegetables: artichokes, 166; as 5-Piece
    Puzzle piece, 90, 150, 151, 185; how to
    use in meals, 90, 150, 151, 164–67
vegetarian meals: weight loss and, 199–201;
    yogurt substitutions for, 30, 50
veggie wraps, 266
Very Berry Omelet with Avocado
    Toast, 101

vinegars, 70, 75–77, 182
vitamin A, 38, 40, 174
vitamin B, 42
vitamin C, 43–44, 77–78, 79, 161
vitamin D, 174, 258–59
vitamin E, 42, 174
vitamin K, 174

walking: afterburn myth and, 247;
    appreciating the beauty of, 236–39;
    finding the time for, 242–47; four unique
    benefits of, 239–42; getting inspired to
    start, 248; health benefits of, 235–36;
    proper footwear for, 242
water intake, 34
weight loss: carbohydrate-protein ratio
    and, 207–9; carb-rich foods and, 170,
    198–99; diet chaos of, 6–7, 9, 10; green
    tea for, 22, 31; impact of antioxidants on,
    74–75; nutrient balance as key to, 196–
    98; organic foods and, 201–7; paying off
    debt metaphor for, 116; processed foods
    impact on, 209–12; regular meals for,
    192–93; studies on almonds and, 41–42;
    studies on naringenin and, 78–79;
    vegetarian meals and, 199–201; vinegar's
    properties for, 75–77; water and, 34. *See
    also* calories; metabolism
weight-loss questions: on bloating, 254–55;
    on falling off track, 253–54; on helping
    husband to lose weight, 256–57; on
    liposuction and plastic surgery, 255–56;
    on weight fluctuation, 249–50; why
    different people lose weight faster, 250,
    253. *See also* personal health questions

whole grains: as 5-Piece Puzzle piece, 90,
    150, 151–52, 185; grocery shopping
    tips on, 263–64; suggestions for using,
    167–71
Wild Rice and Chicken Lettuce Wraps with
    Citrus Slaw, 122
women: fluid requirements of, 34; folate-
    rich foods and colorectal cancer risk of,
    40; health impact of optimism on, 62;
    studies on red meat intake by, 94

Yesism, 228
"Yes!" moments, 1–2, 6
yogurt: California Harvest Pita with
    Minted Yogurt, 102; Cinnamon Cherry
    Yogurt with Peanut Butter Crackers, 115;
    coconut, 30, 50, 51; Dark Chocolate
    Oatmeal with a Side of Minted Blueberry
    Yogurt, 101; 5-Day Fast Forward plan use
    of, 30; Ginger Yogurt with Carambola
    Crunch, 115; grocery guidelines for,
    31, 37, 50–52; nutritional benefits of,
    48–50; Pineapple Almond Peppercorn
    Parfait, 112; Strawberry Vanilla Hazelnut
    "Ice Cream," 110; Strawberry Walnut
    "Ice Cream" with Lime Zest, 114; Vanilla
    Almond Frozen Banana, 115; vegetarian
    and vegan substitutions for, 30, 50

Zero-Prep Cinch! core meal kits, 156–58,
    277–78
Zesty Bean and Summer Slaw Pita, 135
Zesty Cinnamon Basil Berry Tea, 21–22,
    32, 93
Zesty Cranberry Walnut Parfait, 97

# about the author

Cynthia Sass is an award-winning registered dietitian and health educator who has helped millions of Americans fall in love with healthy food. While serving as the nutrition director at *Prevention* magazine, Cynthia created the revolutionary eating plan for Flat Belly Diet!, along with co-authoring the book, which transformed the lives and bellies of women across the globe. In *Cinch!* Cynthia reveals her brand-new cutting-edge strategy for reaching your weight goal while optimizing your health and energy—and it doesn't require counting calories or grams. This flavorful, satisfying plan, which includes a daily dose of dark chocolate, is so easy you'll be able to follow it whether you're cooking at home or dining out.

Cynthia is the real deal. She graduated with highest honors from Syracuse University, where she earned both her bachelor's degree and master's degree in nutrition science. She holds a second master's degree in public health with a focus on community and family health education from the University of South Florida, where she taught in the School of Physical Education and Exercise Science for seven years. In addition to her degrees, Cynthia has completed a personal-training certification and formal culinary training in vegan organic culinary arts. She has almost two decades of experience and is one of America's most sought after health professionals.

Cynthia is a contributing editor and weight-loss columnist for *Shape* magazine and writes for numerous publications, including *More, Good Housekeeping,* and *Reader's Digest.* Cynthia is a contributor and food coach for ABC News and regularly appears on the *Today* show, *The Early Show, Extra!,* and FOX News. She has appeared on *Good Morning America,* the *Rachael Ray Show, The Biggest Loser, The Dr. Oz Show, Nightline,* ABC's *World News,* and many other national television programs.

Cynthia was one of the first dietitians to become board certified as a specialist in sports dietetics by the American Dietetic Association. She has been a nutrition consultant to professional sports teams including the Philadelphia Phillies and Tampa Bay Rays and privately counsels professional and competitive athletes in numerous sports. She is a contributing editor and the exclusive nutritionist for *Athletes Quarterly,* a magazine for current and former professional American athletes.

Through her Manhattan-based private practice, Cynthia counsels a wide range of clients, from celebrities, athletes, and CEOs to teens, men, women, couples, and families. Her specialties include all-natural weight loss, natural and organic nutrition, vegetarian and vegan nutrition, eating for optimal wellness and disease prevention, nutrition for athletes and active people, and overcoming emotional eating. She lives in Manhattan with her husband of thirteen years, Jack Bremen, who has lost over fifty pounds since they met and has kept it off. Cynthia's favorite Cinch! meal is Black Bean Tacos with Cilantro-Jalapeño Guacamole.

## www.cinchyourself.com